I0503656

RENAL DIET
COOKBOOK

Discover which are the main causes of kidney
diseases and how to eat healthy to avoid them
with many renal diet recipes: low sodium, low
potassium, low protein, low calcium and low
phosphorus recipes

TOSHIMORI YOICHI,
MARK DANIEL COOKSEY

Table of Contents

Introduction 8

Definition 8

Components of a renal diet 9

Sodium 9

Potassium 12

Protein 14

Liquids 15

How is a renal diet different? 16

What is renal diet for? 24

Controlling Phosphorous 24

Controlling Potassium 26

Controlling Your Sodium 28

Controlling Your Protein 29

Controlling Your Fluid Intake 30

Fast food facts for the renal patient 31

Dining for the Renal Patient 34

Renal diet on a holiday 36

Renal friendly diets 38

How to be successful on a renal diet 39

Dietary Guidelines for Adults Starting on
Hemodialysis 41

Nutrition and Kidney Disease 60

Diets for Kidney Patients 60

What are kidney diseases and what causes them? 67

Kidney Diseases 67

Symptoms of Kidney diseases 69

Treatment of Kidney Failure 71

Adjusting to Kidney Failure 72

What are kidney diseases 72

Dialysis and kidney ailment 84

More About Kidney Diseases 90

Ten Signs you might be having kidney diseases 93

Why does the renal diet work? 99

Eating Right for Chronic Kidney Disease 99

The subsequent stages to eating right ... 104

What are renal diet benefits? 110

Cardiovascular and renal advantages of dry bean and soybean consumption 114

Benefits of Renal Diet 116

The renal benefits of a healthy life style 118

Easing back the movement of constant renal disappointment: Economic advantages and patients' points of view **136**

What you can eat and what is forbidden in the renal diet **139**

Dull Colored Colas **139**

Avocados **140**

Canned Foods **141**

Entire Wheat Bread **142**

Dark colored Rice **143**

Bananas **144**

Dairy **145**

Oranges and Orange Juice **146**

What to eat in a renal diet? **147**

What you can drink in the renal diet? **149**

Things you can drink **149**

Is liquor or soft drink awful for the kidneys? **150**

Is cranberry squeeze useful for the kidneys? **151**

Shouldn't something be said about caffeinated drinks? **152**

How much water would it be advisable for me to drink? **153**

Recipes 154

Breakfast... 154

Dilly Scrambled Eggs 154

Speedy and Easy Apple Oatmeal Custard
.... 156

Microwave Coffee Cup Egg Scramble
.... 159

Smoothies and drinks........................... 161

Blueberry Smoothie 161

Simple Pineapple Protein Smoothie . 162

Snacks and sides 163

Lunch 166

Bar-b-que Chicken Pita Pizza........... 166

Conclusion.. 169

Introduction

Definition

Individuals images with bargained kidney capacity must stick to a renal or kidney diet to eliminate the measure of waste in their blood. Squanders in the blood originate from nourishment and fluids that are devoured. At the point when kidney capacity is undermined, the kidneys not channel or evacuate squander appropriately. In the event that waste is left in the blood, it can contrarily influence a patient's electrolyte levels. Following a kidney diet may likewise help advance kidney work and moderate the movement of complete kidney disappointment.

A renal eating routine is one that is low in sodium, phosphorous, and protein. A renal eating regimen additionally accentuates the significance of expending top notch protein and typically restricting liquids. A few patients may likewise need to restrain potassium and calcium. Each individual's body is unique, and along these lines, it is vital that every patient works with a renal dietitian work to think of an eating routine that is customized to the patient's needs.

The following are a few substances that are pivotal to screen to advance a renal eating routine:

Components of a renal diet

Sodium

What is Sodium and its job in the body?

Sodium is a mineral found in most characteristic nourishments. The vast majority consider salt and sodium as tradable. Salt, be that as it may, is really a compound of sodium and chloride. Nourishments we eat may contain salt or they may contain sodium in different structures. Handled nourishments frequently contain more significant levels of sodium due to included salt. Sodium is one of the body's three significant electrolytes (potassium and chloride are the other two). Electrolytes control the liquids going all through the body's tissues and cells. Sodium adds to:

Directing circulatory strain and blood volume

Directing nerve capacity and muscle compression

Directing the corrosive base equalization of blood

Adjusting how much liquid the body keeps or dispenses with

For what reason should kidney patients screen sodium admission?

An excessive amount of sodium can be unsafe for individuals with kidney malady in light of the fact that their kidneys can't sufficiently wipe out abundance sodium and liquid from the body. As sodium and liquid develop in the tissues and circulation system, they may cause:

Expanded thirst

Edema: growing in the legs, hands, and face

Hypertension

Cardiovascular breakdown: overabundance liquid in the circulatory system can exhaust your heart, making it developed and powerless

Brevity of breath: liquid can develop in the lungs, making it hard to relax

In what capacity would patients be able to screen their sodium consumption?

Continuously read nourishment marks. Sodium substance is constantly recorded.

Give close consideration to serving sizes.

Utilize crisp, instead of bundled meats.

Pick crisp leafy foods or no-salt-included canned and solidified produce.

Stay away from handled nourishments.

Look at brands and use things that are most minimal in sodium.

Use flavors that don't list "salt" in their title (pick garlic powder rather than garlic salt.)

Cook at home and don't include salt.

Cutoff all out sodium substance to 400 mg for each supper and 150 mg for each tidbit.

Printable Low Sodium Diet Guidelines

Potassium

What is Potassium and its job in the body?

Potassium is a mineral found in a significant number of the nourishments we eat and is likewise found normally in the body. Potassium assumes a job in keeping the heartbeat standard and the muscles working accurately. Potassium is additionally essential for keeping up liquid and electrolyte balance in the circulatory system. The kidneys help to keep the perfect measure of potassium in your body and they oust abundance sums into the pee.

For what reason should kidney patients screen their potassium admission?

At the point when the kidneys come up short, they can never again evacuate abundance potassium, so potassium levels develop in the body. High potassium in the blood is called hyperkalemia which can cause:

Muscle shortcoming

A sporadic heart beat

Slow heartbeat

Respiratory failures

Demise

In what capacity would patients be able to screen their potassium consumption?

At the point when the kidneys never again control potassium, a patient must screen the measure of potassium that enters the body.

High-potassium-food Tips to help keep the degrees of potassium in your blood safe, try to:

Converse with a renal dietitian about making an eating plan.

Breaking point nourishments that are high in potassium.

Breaking point milk and dairy items to 8 oz every day.

Pick crisp foods grown from the ground.

Stay away from salt substitutes and seasonings with potassium.

Peruse marks on bundled nourishments and stay away from potassium chloride.

Give close consideration to serving size.

Keep a nourishment diary.

Protein

Protein isn't an issue for solid kidneys. Typically, protein is ingested and squander items are made, which thus are separated by the nephrons of the kidney. At that point, with the assistance of extra renal proteins, the waste transforms into pee. Conversely, harmed kidneys neglect to expel protein waste and it gathers in the blood. The best possible utilization of protein is precarious for Chronic Kidney Disease patients as the sum contrasts with each phase of ailment. Protein is fundamental for tissue support and other substantial jobs, so it is critical to eat the prescribed sum for the particular phase of malady as per your nephrologist or renal dietician.

Liquids

Liquid control is significant for patients in the later phases of Chronic Kidney Disease since ordinary liquid utilization may cause liquid develop in the body which could wind up hazardous. Individuals on dialysis regularly have diminished pee yield, so expanded liquid in the body can put superfluous weight on the individual's heart and lungs. A patient's liquid stipend is determined on an individual premise, contingent upon pee yield and dialysis settings. It is essential to pursue your nephrologist's/nutritionist's liquid admission rules.

To control liquid admission, patients should:

Not drink more than what your primary care physician orders

Tally all nourishments that will liquefy at room temperature (Jell-O®, popsicles, and so on.)

Be mindful of the measure of liquids utilized in cooking

How is a renal diet different?

At the point when your kidneys are not filling in just as they should, waste and liquid develop in your body. After some time, the waste and additional liquid can reason heart, bone and other medical issues. A kidney-accommodating supper plan restricts the amount of specific minerals and liquid you eat and drink. This can help shield the waste and liquid from structure up and causing issues. How exacting your supper plan ought to be relies upon your phase of kidney ailment. In the beginning periods of kidney malady, you may have almost no cutoff points on what you eat and drink. As your kidney sickness deteriorates, your primary care physician may suggest that you limit:

Potassium

Phosphorus

Liquids

Potassium is a mineral found in practically all nourishments. Your body needs some potassium to make your muscles work, however an excess of potassium can be perilous. At the point when your kidneys are not functioning admirably, your potassium level might be excessively high or excessively low. Having excessively or too little potassium can cause muscle spasms, issues with the manner in which your heart thumps and muscle shortcoming. On the off chance that you have kidney sickness, you may need to constrain how a lot of potassium you take in. Ask your primary care physician or dietitian on the off chance that you have to restrict potassium. Utilize the rundown beneath to realize which nourishments are low or high in potassium. Your dietitian can likewise assist you with figuring out how to securely eat modest quantities of your preferred nourishments that are high in potassium.

Eat this ... (lower-potassium nourishments)

Apples, cranberries, grapes, pineapples and strawberries

Cauliflower, onions, peppers, radishes, summer squash, lettuce

Pita, tortillas and white breads

Meat and chicken, white rice

Instead of ... (higher-potassium nourishments)

Avocados, bananas, melons, oranges, prunes and raisins

Artichokes, winter squash, plantains, spinach, potatoes and tomatoes

Grain items and granola

Beans (prepared, dark, pinto, and so on.), darker or wild rice

Your primary care physician may likewise guide you to take an exceptional drug called a potassium folio to enable your body to dispose of additional potassium.

Get familiar with high potassium and its treatment here

Phosphorus

Phosphorus is a mineral found in practically all nourishments. It works with calcium and nutrient D to keep your bones solid. Solid kidneys keep the perfect measure of phosphorus in your body. At the point when your kidneys are not functioning admirably, phosphorus can develop in your blood. A lot of phosphorus in your blood can prompt powerless bones that break effectively.

Numerous individuals with kidney infection need to restrict phosphorus. Inquire as to whether you have to restrain phosphorus.

Contingent upon your phase of kidney infection, your primary care physician may likewise endorse a medication called a phosphate folio. This shields phosphorus from working up in your blood. A phosphate folio can be useful, yet you will in any case need to observe how a lot of phosphorus you eat. Inquire as to whether a phosphate folio is directly for you. Utilize the rundown beneath to get a few thoughts regarding how to settle on sound decisions on the off chance that you have to restrain phosphorus.

Eat this ... (lower-phosphorous nourishments)

Italian, French or sourdough bread

Corn or rice grains and cream of wheat

Unsalted popcorn

Some light-shaded soft drinks and lemonade

Instead of ... (higher-phosphorous nourishments)

Entire grain bread

Grain oats and oats

Nuts and sunflower seeds

Dull shaded colas

Liquids

You need water to live, yet when you have kidney malady, you may not require to such an extent. This is on the grounds that harmed kidneys don't dispose of additional liquid just as they should. An excessive amount of liquid in your body can be hazardous. It can cause hypertension, expanding and cardiovascular breakdown. Additional liquid can likewise develop around your lungs and make it difficult to relax.

Contingent upon your phase of kidney infection and your treatment, your primary care physician may guide you to constrain liquid. In the event that your primary care physician discloses to you this, you should reduce the amount you drink. You may likewise need to decrease a few nourishments that contain a ton of water. Soups or nourishments that dissolve, similar to ice, dessert and gelatin, have a great deal of water. Numerous products of the soil are high in water, as well. Ask your primary care physician or dietitian in the event that you have to confine liquids.

On the off chance that you do need to restrict liquids, measure your liquids and drink from little cups to assist you with monitoring the amount you've needed to drink. Limit sodium to assist cut with bringing down on thirst. On occasion, you may at present feel parched. To help extinguish your thirst, you may attempt to:

Bite gum

Flush your mouth

Suck on a bit of ice, mints or hard treat (Remember to pick sans sugar sweets in the event that you have diabetes. Squanders in the blood originate from nourishment and fluids that are expended. Individuals with kidney malady must hold fast to a renal eating regimen to eliminate the measure of waste in their blood. Following a renal eating regimen may likewise support kidney capacity and defer complete kidney disappointment. A renal eating regimen is one that is low in sodium, phosphorous and protein. A renal eating regimen focuses on the significance of expending top notch protein and constraining liquids. Some renal weight control plans may likewise call for constrained potassium and calcium. Each individual is extraordinary, and along these lines, a dietician will work with every patient to think of a renal eating routine that is custom-made to their needs.

What is renal diet for?

A renal diet is for the control of successive elements in your body in order to regulate a firm metabolism in yourself.

Controlling Phosphorous

Phosphorus is a mineral that sound kidneys get free of in the pee. In kidneys that are coming up short, phosphorus develops in the blood and may cause numerous issues counting muscle a throbbing painfulness, fragile, effectively broken bones, calcification of the heart, skin, joints, and blood vessels. To hold your phosphorus levels under wraps, think about the accompanying tips:

1. Breaking point high phosphorus nourishments, for example,

• Meats, poultry, dairy and fish (you ought to have 1 serving of 7-8

ounces)

• Milk and other dairy items like cheddar (you ought to have

one 4 oz. serving)

2. Stay away from high phosphorus nourishments, for example,

• Lima Beans, Black Beans, Red Beans, Black-looked at Peas, White

Beans, and Garbanzo Beans

• Dark, entire or grungy grains

 Refrigerator batters like Pillsbury

• Dried vegetables and natural products

• Chocolate

• Dark shaded soft drinks

3. Remember to take your phosphate fasteners with dinners and tidbits.

• Your primary care physician will endorse a prescription called a phosphate fastener which will be some kind of polymer gel or calcium prescription. You have to accept your phosphate folio as endorsed by your primary care physician. Regularly you will take a phosphate folio with each supper and tidbit.

4. Typically you're eating routine is restricted to 1000 mg of phosphorus for each day

Controlling Potassium

Potassium is a component that is essential for the body to keep a typical water balance between the cells and body liquids. All nourishments contain some potassium; however, some contain bigger sums. Ordinary kidney capacity will evacuate potassium through pee. Kidneys that are not working appropriately can't expel the potassium in the pee, so it develops in the blood. This can be exceptionally perilous to your heart. High potassium can cause unpredictable heart thumps and can even reason the heart to stop if the potassium levels get to high. Normally, there are no side effects for somebody with a high potassium level. In the event that you are worried about your potassium level, check with your PCP, and pursue the tips underneath.

• Usually a renal patient's eating routine ought to be constrained to 2000 mg of potassium every day.

• The accompanying nourishments are high in potassium:

Bananas Avocado Oranges

Squeezed orange Prunes Prune Juice

Tomatoes Tomato Juice Tomato Sauce

Melon Tomato Puree Honeydew Melon

Nuts Papaya Chocolate

Red Beans Milk White Beans

Lima Beans Garbanzo Beans Black Beans

Lentils Split peas Baked Beans

Exceptionally Prepared Potatoes:

1. Strip and cut into 1/8 inch pieces.

2. Absorb 1 cup potatoes 5 cups of water for 2 hours.

3. Channel and flush and channel.

4. Cook in a lot of water.

5. Channel and pound, fry or serve plain.

Controlling Your Sodium

Sodium, or sodium chloride, is a component that is utilized by every living animal to control the water content in the body. Generally a sodium confinement comes in the type of "No Added Salt." This is important in light of the fact that a more noteworthy admission of sodium will result in inadequately controlled circulatory strain and over the top thirst which can prompt trouble holding fast to the liquid confinements in your eating regimen.

To confine your sodium, you should:

• Avoid table salt and any seasonings that end with "salt"

• Avoid salt substitutes (they contain potassium)

• Avoid salty meats, for example, bacon, ham, frankfurter, sausages, lunch meats, canned meats, or bologna

• Avoid salty snacks, for example, cheddar twists, salted saltines, nuts, and chips

• Avoid canned soups, solidified meals, and moment noodles

• Avoid packaged sauces, pickles, olives, and MSG

Controlling Your Protein

Protein is essential to help in development and upkeep of body tissue. Protein likewise plays a job in battling contamination, recuperating of wounds, and gives a wellspring of vitality to the body.

- You should make a point to eat 7-8 ounces of protein consistently. Nourishments that are high in protein incorporate hamburger, pork, veal, chicken, turkey, fish, fish, and eggs.

- 1 egg is equivalent to 1 ounce of protein, and three ounces of protein is practically identical to the size of a deck of cards.

Controlling Your Fluid Intake

Individuals on dialysis regularly have diminished pee yield, so expanded liquid in the body can put pointless pressure on the individual's heart and lungs.

- A liquid remittance for singular patients is determined based on 'pee in addition to 500ml.' The 500 ml covers the loss of liquids through the skin and lungs.

- Most patients won't pee as much once they start Hemodialysis.

The individuals who produce a great deal of pee might have the option to drink more than those who don't deliver pee.

• Between every dialysis treatment, patients are relied upon to increase a little weight because of the water content in nourishments (leafy foods).

• The measure of liquid in a run of the mill day's feast (barring liquids, for example, water, tea, and so forth.) is in any event 500 ml and subsequently anticipated day by day weight

addition is between 0.4 – 0.5kg.

• To control liquid admission, patients should:

☐ Not drink more than what your primary care physician orders (normally 4 cups of liquid every day)

☐ Count all nourishments that will liquefy at room temperature (Jell-O® , popsicles, and natural product frosts).

Fast food facts for the renal patient

Fast help eateries give us a speedy, simple, modest chomp when we're in a hurry. Americans love inexpensive food and there are such a significant number of things to browse! A ton of chains are presently advertising lower-fat choices and whenever picked admirably, quick nourishments can be solid AND fit into your renal eating routine. On the off chance that you are a customary through the drive-up window or much of the time eat in at drive-through joints, keep these tips as a main priority.

Some Ordering Tips:

• Burgers and sandwiches are high in sodium since they are pre-salted. This might be troublesome for the brisk help eatery to discard the salt. Make certain to ask before you request.

• Remember that fries and heated potatoes are wealthy in potassium. In any case, in the event that you can't envision a burger without the fries, request a little serving and request unsalted, if conceivable.

• Keep as a main priority that catsup, mustard, and pickles are for the most part high in sodium. Keep toppings, uncommon sauces and dressings to a base. Solicitation that these garnishes be served "as an afterthought" so you can control the sum.

• Beverage measures commonly are enormous or "super-size" and can add to liquid over-burden if the whole drink is devoured. Request a little drink and make certain to consider it part of your liquid stipend.

• Balance inexpensive food things with other nourishment decisions. As you request, think about different nourishments you have eaten or will eat during the day.

• Choose cooked, steamed or barbecued things over profound fat seared nourishments. To cut back the excess from seared things, request the customary assortment rather than the extra firm and evacuate the skin before eating. Evacuating the skin likewise brings down the sodium content since most hitters and coatings normally incorporate seasonings wealthy in sodium. The immense assortment of vegetables and natural products can give you nutrients An and C, folic corrosive and fiber. Be cautious however, an excursion to the plate of mixed greens bar can furnish you with more fat and calories than a hamburger and French fries! There are numerous serving of mixed greens bar things that can without much of a stretch fit into your renal eating routine.

Dining for the Renal Patient

Eating out in eateries can be troublesome when you are on dialysis. A few amazing assets are found in the NFK Publication "Feasting Out with Certainty." If you have a most loved eatery, approach the administrator for a duplicate of the menu to take to your unit dietitian and they can assist you with making great decisions.

Italian Food

Italian eateries offer a great deal of things appropriate for the renal eating routine. The stunt here is to request the sauce as an afterthought. The red based sauces have potassium and the white sauces are high in phosphorus. You can differ the sauces and the kinds of pasta to make fascinating dinners. Pesto sauce is garlic, basil and oil and is a decent other option. Some shellfish and mussel sauces are not tomato or on the other hand cream-based and are great decisions for fish sweethearts. Plates of mixed greens and breads are incredible decisions here; simply request no olives and cheddar. Keep in mind to request the dressing as an afterthought.

It is smarter to keep away from the dishes like lasagna, cannelloni, ravioli and comparable things as they contain high sodium, high potassium, and high phosphorus fixings. Generally Italian eateries additionally offer some sort of flame broiled chicken as an option to their pasta dish. Have the chicken, serving of mixed greens and bread for your dinner and take the pasta home and have with your claim bread and plate of mixed greens for lunch the following day.

Asian Restaurants

These are troublesome spots to eat in light of the high sodium substance. Chinese cafés are the most troublesome in light of the enormous number of blended dishes in with soy, hoisin, and prepared sauces. They all contain salt as well as MSG. Thai nourishments by and large have more flavors and less sodium, habitually you can request sauces as an afterthought. Japanese cafés will likewise serve more spiced nourishments and cook less with sodium.

Renal diet on a holiday

You can have a pleasant Christmas season this year on the off chance that you settle on the correct decisions. Numerous conventional top choices contain an excessive amount of potassium for renal patients. This article will appear you how to appreciate the special seasons without feeling severely or trying too hard. Browse the Occasion Food list beneath.

Hors d'oeuvres

Celery and Carrot Sticks with cream cheddar

Bagel Chips-Unsalted

Bread Sticks

Cream Cheese or Sour Cream and Dill Dip

Chicken Wings (No Salt Added)

Mixed drink Meatballs (No Salt Added)

Wafers Unsalted

Deviled Eggs

Characteristic Tortilla Chips-Unsalted

Popcorn

Pretzels-Unsalted

Shrimp

Renal friendly diets

On the off chance that your primary care physician has endorsed liquor, maintain a strategic distance from high potassium beverages, for example, ridiculous mary's, screw drivers and pina coladas.

◆Go simple on salty nourishments. It will help you from getting parched time and again.

◆For the primary course, pick new, natural meats like capon, hamburger or pork. Maintain a strategic distance from ham and selfbasting turkeys due to the unnecessary sodium.

◆Substitute rice or an additional aiding of stuffing for potatoes to decrease the potassium in your dinner.

◆Remember to check Jell-O® or Jell-O® servings of mixed greens as a major aspect of your treats.

◆Use whipped cream rather than frozen yogurt on treats.

◆If you have a huge feast, go simple on what you eat the following day. Take your phosphate covers with or following the supper.

How to be successful on a renal diet

Balance

The Dietary Guidelines for Americans accentuates the significance of eating a assortment of nourishments. This applies to dialysis patients, as well. You can appreciate all nourishments in balance while following a renal eating regimen. One of the rules states: "Be reasonable: Enjoy all nourishments, simply don't try too hard."

We Encourage You To:

• Slow down while eating. It takes 20 minutes to send the sign that you've had enough to eat.

• Stop eating when full. Patients should leave the table inclination that they can eat somewhat more.

• Have one little aiding of that chocolate cake and appreciate each chomp.

• Enjoy that bit of lasagna twice to such an extent. Eat half in the café and take the rest home to appreciate the following day.

The Goal

The objective for our patients ought to be a solid way of life that can be kept up as opposed to a transient eating regimen that will in all probability be deserted and produce mental uneasiness.

Diet - ceaseless kidney malady

You may need to cause changes to your eating regimen when you to have interminable kidney infection (CKD). These progressions may incorporate restricting liquids, eating a low-protein diet, constraining salt, potassium, phosphorous, and different electrolytes, and getting enough calories on the off chance that you are shedding pounds. You may need to change your eating regimen more if your kidney malady deteriorates, or in the event that you need dialysis.

Capacity

The reason for this eating routine is to keep the degrees of electrolytes, minerals, and liquid in your body adjusted when you have CKD or are on dialysis. Individuals on dialysis need this uncommon eating routine to constrain the development of waste items in the body. Restricting liquids between dialysis medicines is significant on the grounds that a great many people on dialysis pee practically nothing. Without pee, liquid will develop in the body and cause an excess of liquid in the heart and lungs.

Dietary Guidelines for Adults Starting on Hemodialysis

Since you are starting hemodialysis, there might be numerous adjustments in your day by day life. Your primary care physician has likely disclosed to you that you may need to roll out certain improvements in your eating regimen.

How well you feel will rely upon:

Eating the correct kind and measures of nourishment.

Having the hemodialysis medications your wellbeing expert requests for you

Taking the meds your wellbeing expert requests for you.

Your eating regimen is a significant piece of your treatment. Your kidneys can't dispose of enough waste items and liquids from your blood and your body presently has unique needs. Along these lines, you should confine liquids and change your admission of specific nourishments in your eating regimen. The kidney dietitian at your dialysis focus will assist you with arranging an eating regimen for your uncommon needs.

Utilize this pamphlet as a guide until your dietitian readies a customized feast plan for you. You should:

Eat all the higher protein nourishments.

Eat less high salt, high potassium, and high phosphorus nourishments.

Figure out how much liquid you can securely drink (counting espresso, tea, water, and any nourishment that is fluid at room temperature).

Salt and Sodium

Utilize less salt and eat less salty nourishments: This may control circulatory strain. It might likewise help lessen liquid weight gains between dialysis sessions since salt builds thirst and makes the body hold (or clutch) liquid.

Use herbs, flavors, and low-salt flavor enhancers instead of salt

Keep away from salt substitutes made with potassium.

Meat/Protein

Individuals on dialysis need to eat more protein. Protein can help keep sound blood protein levels and improve wellbeing. Protein additionally helps keep your muscles solid, assists wounds with mending quicker, reinforces your safe framework, and improves generally wellbeing. Eat a high protein nourishment (meat, fish, poultry, crisp pork, or eggs) at each dinner, or around 8-10 ounces of high protein nourishments consistently.

3 ounces = the size of a deck of cards, a medium pork hack, a ¼ pound burger patty, ½ chicken bosom, a medium fish filet.

1 ounce = 1 egg or ¼-cup egg substitute, ¼-cup fish, ¼-cup ricotta cheddar, 1 cut of low sodium lunchmeat, 1tablespoon nutty spread, ½ ounce of nuts or seeds

Note: Even however nutty spread, nuts, seeds, dried beans, peas, and lentils have protein, these nourishments are commonly constrained in light of the fact that they are high in both potassium and phosphorus.

Grains/Cereals/Bread

Except if you have to confine your calorie admission for weight reduction and additionally oversee starch consumption for glucose control, you may eat, as you want from this nutrition class. Grains, oats, and breads are a decent wellspring of calories. A great many people need 6 - 11 servings from this gathering every day.

Sums equivalent to one serving:

1 cut bread (white, rye, or sourdough)

½ English biscuit

½ bagel

½ cheeseburger bun

½ frank bun

1 6-inch tortilla

½ cup cooked pasta

½ cup cooked white rice

½ cup cooked oat (like cream of wheat)

1 cup cold oat (like corn drops or fresh rice)

4 unsalted saltines

1½ cups unsalted popcorn

10 vanilla wafers

Maintain a strategic distance from "entire grain" and "high fiber" nourishments (like entire wheat bread, wheat oat and dark colored rice) to assist you with constraining your admission of phosphorus. By constraining dairy–based nourishments you secure your bones and veins.

Milk/Yogurt/Cheese

Point of confinement your admission of milk, yogurt, and cheddar to ½-cup milk or ½-cup yogurt or 1-ounce cheddar every day. Most dairy nourishments are high in phosphorus.

The phosphorus substance is the equivalent for a wide range of milk – skim, low fat, and entirety! On the off chance that you do eat any high-phosphorus nourishments, take a phosphate cover with that supper.

Dairy nourishments "low" in phosphorus:

(get some information about the serving size that is directly for you)

Spread and tub margarine

Cream cheddar

Substantial cream

Ricotta cheddar

Brie cheddar

Non-dairy whipped beating

Sherbet

On the off chance that you have or are in danger for coronary illness, a portion of the high fat nourishments recorded above may not be great decisions for you.

Certain brands of non-dairy creams and "milk, (for example, rice milk) are low in phosphorus and potassium. Approach your dietitian for subtleties.

Organic product/Juice

All organic products have some potassium, however certain natural products have more than others and ought to be constrained or completely dodged. Constraining potassium ensures your heart.

Breaking point or evade :

Oranges and squeezed orange

Kiwis

Nectarines

Prunes and prune juice

Raisins and dried organic product

Bananas

Melons (melon and honeydew)

Continuously AVOID star organic product (carambola).

Eat 2-3 servings of low potassium organic products every day.

One serving = ½-cup or 1 little organic product or 4 ounces of juice.

Pick:

Apple (1)

Berries (½ cup)

Fruits (10)

Organic product mixed drink, depleted (½ cup)

Grapes (15)

Peach (1 little crisp or canned, depleted)

Pear, crisp or canned, depleted (1 divide)

Pineapple (½ cup canned, depleted)

Plums (1-2)

Tangerine (1)

Watermelon (1 little wedge)

Beverages:

Apple juice

Cranberry juice mixed drink

Grape juice

Lemonade

Vegetables/Salads

All vegetables have some potassium, yet certain vegetables have more than others and ought to be restricted or completely dodged. Constraining potassium admission ensures your heart.

Eat 2-3 servings of low-potassium vegetables every day. One serving = ½-cup.

Pick:

Broccoli (crude or cooked from solidified)

Cabbage

Carrots

Cauliflower

Celery

Cucumber

Eggplant

Garlic

Green and Wax beans ("string beans")

Lettuce-different types (1 cup)

Onion

Peppers-different types and hues

Radishes

Watercress

Zucchini and Yellow squash

Point of confinement or stay away from:

Potatoes (counting French Fries, potato chips and sweet potatoes)

Tomatoes and tomato sauce

Winter squash

Pumpkin

Asparagus (cooked)

Avocado

Beets

Beet greens

Cooked spinach

Parsnips and rutabaga

Treat

Contingent upon your calorie needs, your dietitian may prescribe unhealthy deserts. Pies, treats, sherbet, and cakes are great decisions (yet limit dairy-based pastries and those made with chocolate, nuts, and bananas). On the off chance that you have diabetes, examine low sugar dessert decisions with your dietitian.

Test Menu

Breakfast

Cranberry Juice, 4 ounces

Eggs (2) or ½-cup egg substitute

Toasted white or entire wheat bread (2 cuts)

Spread or tub margarine or organic product spread

Espresso, 6 ounces

Lunch

Fish plate of mixed greens sandwich made with 3 ounces fish on a hard move with lettuce and mayonnaise.

(Other great decisions for sandwiches incorporate egg and chicken serving of mixed greens, lean meal meat, low salt ham and turkey bosom.)

Coleslaw, ½-cup

Pretzels (low salt)

Canned and depleted peaches, ½-cup

Soda, 8 ounces

(Cola beverages are high in phosphorus. Pick soda or lemon-lime drinks.)

Supper

Burger patty, 4 ounces on a bun with 1-2 teaspoons ketchup

Plate of mixed greens (1 cup): lettuce, cucumber, radishes, peppers, with olive oil and vinegar dressing

Lemonade, 8 ounces

Go for at any rate 2-3 "fish" dinners every week. Many fish are wealthy in heart-sound "omega-3" fats. Fish and salmon (washed or canned without salt) and shellfish are magnificent heart sound protein decisions.

Tidbit/Dessert

Milk, 4 ounces

Cut of crusty fruit-filled treat

This supper plan gives 2150 Calories, 91 grams protein, 2300 mg sodium, 1800 mg potassium, 950 mg phosphorus. 38 liquid ounces.

In what manner will I know whether I am eating right to remain sound?

Eating admirably causes you remain solid. Eating ineffectively can expand your odds of sickness and influence how you feel. Your dietitian will chat with you about how well you are eating and will assist you with changing your eating regimen to your individual needs dependent on your lab report and discussions with you.

A few inquiries you may be posed:

Have you seen an adjustment in the sort or measure of nourishment you eat every day?

Have you had any issues eating your typical or suggested diet?

Have you shed pounds easily?

Have you seen any adjustments in your quality or capacity to deal with yourself?

Your dietitian or medical attendant may take a gander at the fat and muscle stores in your face, hands, arms, shoulders, and legs. Your dialysis care group will search for changes in your blood level of proteins, and particularly one called "egg whites." An adjustment in this protein can imply that you are losing body protein, yet egg whites can likewise be influenced on the off chance that you have a contamination or are putting on an excessive amount of liquid load between medications. The dietitian may prescribe a protein supplement, for example, Nepro™ or LiquaCel™ to expand protein levels. The dietitian may likewise recommend little incessant dinners and bites. Work with your dietitian to improve your blood level of protein. The perfect measure of dialysis is likewise significant for eating great and remaining solid.

Imagine a scenario in which I have elevated cholesterol.

Changing your eating routine may help bring down the cholesterol level in your blood. Your dietitian will converse with you about the sorts of fat and creature nourishments you eat. Expanding admission of low potassium products of the soil, diminishing the measure of seared nourishments, notwithstanding 150 minutes of physical action every week can improve cholesterol levels. Imagine a scenario where I have diabetes.

From the start the kidney and diabetic eating regimen give off an impression of being altogether different, however they are similar from numerous points of view. The two weight control plans suggest eating 3 adjusted suppers, evading a lot of protein, and restricting sodium. A fair supper has in any event 3 of the nutrition classes (protein, grain, vegetables, natural products, and dairy). The kidney diet confines the measure of milk that you drink, yet numerous individuals with diabetes as of now limit milk to 4 ounces every day. Both prescribe ½ plate of vegetables, ¼ plate of starch rich nourishment, ¼ plate of high protein nourishment, and a bit of organic product. The greatest change is that the kidney diet doesn't have as a lot of assortment in the kinds of foods grown from the ground decisions since some have more potassium than others. The diabetic eating routine prescribes 45 to 75 grams of sugar with every feast and dispersing suppers 4 to 5 hours separated. This suggestion is useful for the kidney diet, as well. Both the kidney and diabetic eating routine assistance to keep your heart solid.

Now and again, you may need to make just a couple of changes in your eating routine to meet your requirements as a kidney quiet. For instance, you may need to constrain a portion of the free nourishments you have been utilizing may should be restricted on your kidney diet. Your dietitian will help make a feast arrangement particularly for you.

Is there something else I should know?

The accompanying significant hints can be useful with your eating regimen:

Crisp or plain solidified vegetables contain no additional salt. Channel all the cooking fluid before serving.

Canned organic products generally contain less potassium than crisp natural products. Channel all the fluid before serving.

Rice and almond milk are low in phosphorus and can be utilized instead of milk.

Marks on nourishment bundles will give you data about a portion of the fixings that may not be permitted in your eating regimen. Figure out how to peruse these marks to assist you with restricting sodium and control phosphorous. Maintain a strategic distance from nourishments with fixings that contain "PHOS"

To assist you with maintaining a strategic distance from salt, numerous herbs and flavors can be utilized to make your eating regimen all the more intriguing. Check with your dietitian for a rundown of these.

Nutrition and Kidney Disease

Most patients in the beginning times of kidney malady need to confine the measure of sodium in their eating regimen. A few patients might be advised to restrain protein in their eating routine too. The DASH diet is frequently suggested for patients with kidney malady. Make certain to converse with your social insurance supplier about your particular sustenance needs.

Diets for Kidney Patients

Dealing with your eating routine with kidney sickness

When living with constant kidney sickness, overseeing what you eat and drink can be a test; notwithstanding, your eating regimen can likewise emphatically impact how you feel, and what different medications you may require. An Accredited Practicing Dietitian experienced in kidney sickness, called a Renal Dietitian, is the best individual to counsel about an individualized feast plan. The initial step will be a dietary appraisal to survey your admission of vitality and significant supplements.

Dietary appraisal incorporates an audit of your admission of vitality and significant supplements, for example,

protein

sodium/salt

potassium

phosphate

liquid

fat

Dietary guidance is given on an individual premise, considering what you like to eat, how you are feeling, your age, way of life, weight, muscle size, wellbeing status and blood test outcomes.

Everybody should constrain their salt, sugar and fat admission as a feature of solid living.

As kidney malady advances, your dietary needs are probably going to change. Your kidneys will turn out to be less compelling at evacuating undesirable liquid and dealing with the right degrees of supplements, for example, calcium, phosphate and potassium. The underlying dietary changes prescribed may be little, yet as your kidney malady advances increasingly critical changes might be required. View our scope of diet and sustenance reality sheets here or perceive how to perceive how to decrease your salt admission here.

In the event that you are now on dialysis, see other valuable eating routine and nourishment tips accessible here. Step by step instructions to capitalize on your meeting with a Renal Dietitian

Over various days before your arrangement, record what you eat and take the rundown with you.

Take a rundown of your drugs.

In the event that another person regularly cooks for you, request that they go with you.

Pose inquiries with the goal that you feel sure about what you have to do and why.

Arrange normal follow-up arrangements to screen your advancement.

The Dietitians Association of Australia can give names and contact subtleties of nearby renal dietitians

Keeping up a sound weight

A few people with incessant kidney infection don't want to eat or experience issues eating enough nourishment to remain sound. Unhealthiness can create when nourishment admission is deficient and your body doesn't get the perfect measure of the nutrients, minerals and different supplements. This is increasingly normal in the later phases of incessant kidney malady.

On the off chance that you are getting thinner that isn't arranged, or have any worries about your eating regimen, tell your primary care physician or renal dietitian. Weight increase can likewise cause genuine medical issues. On the off chance that you are overweight it tends to be more diligently to get entrance for dialysis, and you may likewise not be reasonable for a kidney transplant. On the off chance that weight increase is an issue, your renal dietitian can assist you with arranging a fitting eating program. Prior to taking any dietary enhancements or beginning an arrangement to lose or build weight reduction, consistently look for guidance from your primary care physician or renal dietitian. Changes to your nourishment and liquid admission might be not kidding and cause huge harm.

Tips on nutrients and minerals

In case you're not getting every one of the nutrients and minerals you need from the nourishments you eat, at that point nutrient and mineral enhancements might be suggested or endorsed by your PCP or dietitian, contingent upon the phase of your kidney ailment. Normally a well-adjusted eating routine will supply you with enough nutrients and minerals to keep you healthy. Be that as it may, dialysis treatment will wash some water-solvent nutrients out of your body.

At the point when you're on dialysis you should just take nutrient enhancements that have been suggested for you, as specific nutrients and minerals can be destructive. It's significant for you to counsel your primary care physician. Nutrients might be helpful to enhance your wellbeing when you have or experience any of the accompanying:

incessantly poor or flighty dietary patterns

diminished hunger, sickness, heaving

taste changes or nourishment abhorrences

unfortunate weight reduction

nourishment weakness

nutrient misfortune during dialysis.

KidneyVital means to enhance the key nutrients and follow components, to assist you with carrying on with a progressively dynamic life. It has been uniquely detailed by kidney masters to give the supplements your body needs and rejects those fixings that could be destructive to your wellbeing. Wholesome attributes of the five fundamental nutritional categories. Check this diagram beneath for the supplements and other critical segments in the fundamental nutritional categories.

What are kidney diseases and what causes them?

Kidney Diseases

By and large, kidney disappointment is brought about by other medical issues that have done lasting harm (hurt) to your kidneys gradually, after some time. At the point when your kidneys are harmed, they may not fill in just as they should. In the event that the harm to your kidneys keeps on deteriorating and your kidneys are less and less ready to carry out their responsibility, you have incessant kidney sickness. Kidney disappointment is the last (most serious) phase of constant kidney malady. This is the reason kidney disappointment is likewise called end-organize renal sickness, or ESRD for short. Diabetes is the most well-known reason for ESRD. Hypertension is the second most normal reason for ESRD. Different issues that can cause kidney disappointment include:

Immune system ailments, for example, lupus and IgA nephropathy

Hereditary ailments (infections you are brought into the world with, for example, polycystic kidney ailment

Nephrotic disorder

Urinary tract issues

Here and there the kidneys can quit working abruptly (inside two days). This kind of kidney disappointment is called intense kidney damage or intense renal disappointment. Regular reasons for intense renal disappointment include:

Respiratory failure

Illicit medication uses and medication misuse

Insufficient blood streaming to the kidneys

Urinary tract issues

This kind of kidney disappointment isn't constantly changeless. Your kidneys may return to typical or practically ordinary with treatment and in the event that you don't have different genuine medical issues. Having one of the medical issues that can prompt kidney disappointment doesn't imply that you will have kidney disappointment. Carrying on with a solid way of life and working with your PCP to control these medical issues can enable your kidneys to work for whatever length of time that conceivable.

Symptoms of Kidney diseases

Incessant kidney infection (CKD) normally deteriorates gradually, and side effects may not show up until your kidneys are gravely harmed. In the late phases of CKD, as you are nearing kidney disappointment (ESRD), you may see side effects that are brought about by waste and additional liquid structure up in your body.

You may see at least one of the accompanying manifestations if your kidneys are starting to come up short:

Tingling

Muscle issues

Queasiness and heaving

Not feeling hungry

Growing in your feet and lower legs

An excess of (pee) or insufficient pee

Issue resting

Issue resting

On the off chance that your kidneys quit working all of a sudden (intense kidney disappointment), you may see at least one of the accompanying indications:

Stomach (tummy) torment

Back torment

The runs

Fever

Nosebleeds

Rash

Retching

Having at least one of any of the manifestations above might be an indication of genuine kidney issues. On the off chance that you see any of these manifestations, you should contact your primary care physician immediately.

Treatment of Kidney Failure

On the off chance that you have kidney disappointment (end-organize renal ailment or ESRD), you will require dialysis or a kidney transplant to live. There is no remedy for ESRD, however numerous individuals live long lives while on dialysis or subsequent to having a kidney transplant.

Adjusting to Kidney Failure

Discovering that you have kidney disappointment can come as a stun, regardless of whether you have known for quite a while that your kidneys were not functioning admirably. Changing your way of life to set aside a few minutes for your medicines can make adapting to this new reality considerably harder. You may need to quit working or find better approaches to work out. You may feel dismal or apprehensive. All isn't lost. You can find support to feel good and have a satisfying life.

What are kidney diseases

The kidneys are a couple of clench hand measured organs situated at the base of the rib confine. There is one kidney on each side of the spine. Kidneys are fundamental to having a sound body. They are for the most part answerable for sifting waste items, overabundance water, and different debasements out of the blood. These poisons are put away in the bladder and afterward expelled during pee. The kidneys additionally direct pH, salt, and potassium levels in the body. They produce hormones that manage circulatory strain and control the creation of red platelets. The kidneys even initiate a type of nutrient D that enables the body to assimilate calcium.

Kidney malady influences roughly 26 million American grown-ups. It happens when your kidneys become harmed and can't play out their capacity. Harm might be brought about by diabetes, hypertension, and different other constant (long haul) conditions. Kidney malady can prompt other medical issues, including powerless bones, nerve harm, and lack of healthy sustenance.

On the off chance that the sickness deteriorates after some time, your kidneys may quit working totally. This implies dialysis will be required to play out the capacity of the kidneys. Dialysis is a treatment that channels and filters the blood utilizing a machine. It can't fix kidney ailment; however, it can drag out your life.

What are the sorts and reasons for kidney sickness?

Constant kidney illness

The most well-known type of kidney illness is incessant kidney infection. Incessant kidney sickness is a long-haul condition that doesn't improve after some time. It's ordinarily brought about by hypertension.

Hypertension is risky for the kidneys since it can press the glomeruli. Glomeruli are the small veins in the kidneys where blood is cleaned. After some time, the expanded weight harms these vessels and kidney capacity starts to decay.

Kidney capacity will in the end weaken to the point where the kidneys can never again play out their activity appropriately. For this situation, an individual would need to go on dialysis. Dialysis sift additional liquid and waste through of the blood. Dialysis can help treat kidney ailment yet it can't fix it. A kidney transplant might be another treatment choice relying upon your conditions.

Diabetes is likewise a significant reason for incessant kidney infection. Diabetes is a gathering of sicknesses that causes high glucose. The expanded degree of sugar in the blood harms the veins in the kidneys after some time. This implies the kidneys can't spotless the blood appropriately. Kidney disappointment can happen when your body winds up over-burden with poisons.

Kidney stones

Kidney stones are another regular kidney issue. They happen when minerals and different substances in the blood take shape in the kidneys, framing strong masses (stones). Kidney stones for the most part leave the body during pee. Passing kidney stones can be very difficult, however they once in a while cause critical issues.

Glomerulonephritis

Glomerulonephritis is an aggravation of the glomeruli. Glomeruli are very little structures inside the kidneys that channel the blood. Glomerulonephritis can be brought about by diseases, drugs, or inherent anomalies (issue that happen during or not long after birth). It frequently shows signs of improvement all alone.

Polycystic kidney ailment

Polycystic kidney ailment is a hereditary issue that causes various pimples (little sacs of liquid) to develop in the kidneys. These pimples can meddle with kidney capacity and cause kidney disappointment. (Note that individual kidney sores are genuinely normal and quite often innocuous. Polycystic kidney ailment is a different, progressively genuine condition.)

Urinary tract diseases

Urinary tract diseases (UTIs) are bacterial contaminations of any piece of the urinary framework. Diseases in the bladder and urethra are the most widely recognized. They are effectively treatable and seldom lead to more medical issues. Be that as it may, whenever left untreated, these diseases can spread to the kidneys and cause kidney disappointment.

What are the side effects of kidney ailment?

Kidney illness is a condition that can without much of a stretch go unnoticed until the manifestations become extreme. The accompanying manifestations are early cautioning signs that you may be creating kidney sickness:

exhaustion

trouble concentrating

issue dozing

poor hunger

muscle cramping

swollen feet/lower legs

puffiness around the eyes in the first part of the day

dry, layered skin

visit pee, particularly late around evening time

Find out additional: Kidney capacity tests »

Serious side effects that could mean your kidney illness is advancing into kidney disappointment include:

queasiness

retching

loss of craving

changes in pee yield

liquid maintenance

sickliness (a reduction in red platelets)

diminished sex drive

abrupt ascent in potassium levels (hyperkalemia)

irritation of the pericardium (liquid filled sac that covers the heart)

What are the hazard factors for creating kidney infection?

Individuals with diabetes have a higher danger of creating kidney infection. Diabetes is the main source of kidney ailment, representing around 44 percent of new cases. You may likewise be bound to get kidney infection in the event that you:

have hypertension

have other relatives with interminable kidney sickness are older are of African, Hispanic, Asian, or American Indian drop

How is kidney infection analyzed?

Your PCP will initially decide if you have a place in any of the high-hazard gatherings. They will at that point run a few tests to check whether your kidneys are working appropriately. These tests may include:

Glomerular filtration rate (GFR)

This test will quantify how well your kidneys are functioning and decide the phase of kidney illness.

Ultrasound or figured tomography (CT) Scan

Ultrasounds and CT sweeps produce clear pictures of your kidneys and urinary tract. The photos enable your PCP to check whether your kidneys are too little or enormous. They can likewise show any tumors or basic issues that might be available.

Kidney biopsy

During a kidney biopsy, your PCP will evacuate a little bit of tissue from your kidney while you're quieted. The tissue test can enable your primary care physician to decide the sort of kidney ailment you have and how a lot of harm has happened.

Pee test

Your primary care physician may demand a pee test to test for egg whites. Egg whites is a protein that can be passed into your pee when your kidneys are harmed.

Blood creatinine test

Creatinine is a waste item. It's discharged into the blood when creatine (a particle put away in muscle) is separated. The degrees of creatinine in your blood will increment if your kidneys aren't working appropriately.

Find out increasingly: Excessive pee around evening time »

How is kidney illness treated?

Treatment for kidney illness normally centers around controlling the basic reason for the ailment. This implies your PCP will assist you with bettering deal with your circulatory strain, glucose, and cholesterol levels. They may utilize at least one of the accompanying techniques to treat kidney malady.

Medications and medicine

Your PCP will either endorse angiotensin-changing over chemical (ACE) inhibitors, for example, lisinopril and ramipril, or angiotensin receptor blockers (ARBs, for example, irbesartan and olmesartan. These are pulse prescriptions that can slow the movement of kidney infection. Your primary care physician may recommend these drugs to safeguard kidney work, regardless of whether you don't have hypertension.

You may likewise be treated with cholesterol drugs, (for example, simvastatin). These prescriptions can diminish blood cholesterol levels and help keep up kidney wellbeing. Contingent upon your indications, your primary care physician may likewise recommend medications to diminish growing and treat paleness (decline in the quantity of red platelets).

Dietary and way of life changes

Making changes to your eating regimen is similarly as significant as taking drug. Embracing a sound way of life can help anticipate a large number of the basic reasons for kidney infection. Your primary care physician may suggest that you:

control diabetes through insulin infusions

cut back on nourishments high in cholesterol

cut back on salt

start a heart-sound eating regimen that incorporates crisp organic products, veggies, entire grains, and low-fat dairy items

limit liquor utilization

stop smoking

increment physical movement

get more fit

Dialysis and kidney ailment

Dialysis is a counterfeit technique for separating the blood. It's utilized when somebody's kidneys have fizzled or are near falling flat. Numerous individuals with late-arrange kidney ailment must go on dialysis for all time or until a giver kidney is found.

There are two sorts of dialysis: hemodialysis and peritoneal dialysis.

Hemodialysis

In hemodialysis, the blood is siphoned through a unique machine that channels out waste items and liquid. Hemodialysis is done at your home or in an emergency clinic or dialysis focus. The vast majority have three sessions for every week, with every session enduring three to five hours. Be that as it may, hemodialysis should likewise be possible in shorter, progressively visit sessions.

A little while before beginning hemodialysis, a great many people will have medical procedure to make an arteriovenous (AV) fistula. An AV fistula is made by associating a corridor and a vein just beneath the skin, regularly in the lower arm. The bigger vein enables an expanded measure of blood to stream consistently through the body during hemodialysis treatment. This implies more blood can be sifted and sanitized. An arteriovenous unite (a circled, plastic cylinder) might be embedded and utilized for a similar reason if a corridor and vein can't be combined.

The most well-known reactions of hemodialysis are low pulse, muscle cramping, and tingling.

Peritoneal dialysis

In peritoneal dialysis, the peritoneum (layer that lines the stomach divider) subs for the kidneys. A cylinder is embedded and used to fill the belly with a liquid called dialysate. Squander items in the blood stream from the peritoneum into the dialysate. The dialysate is then depleted from the midriff.

There are two types of peritoneal dialysis: persistent wandering peritoneal dialysis, where the stomach area is occupied and depleted a few times during the day, and nonstop cycler-helped peritoneal dialysis, which uses a machine to cycle the liquid all through the guts around evening time while the individual rests.

The most widely recognized reactions of peritoneal dialysis are contaminations in the stomach cavity or in the zone where the cylinder was embedded. Opposite symptoms may incorporate weight increase and hernias. A hernia is the point at which the digestive system pushes through a shaky area or tear in the lower stomach divider.

What is the long-haul standpoint for somebody with kidney sickness?

Kidney malady ordinarily doesn't leave once it's analyzed. The most ideal approach to keep up kidney wellbeing is to receive a solid way of life and pursue your primary care physician's recommendation. Kidney illness can deteriorate after some time. It might even prompt kidney disappointment. Kidney disappointment can be perilous whenever left untreated.

Kidney disappointment happens when your kidneys are scarcely working or not working by any stretch of the imagination. This is overseen by dialysis. Dialysis includes the utilization of a machine to channel squander from your blood. At times, your primary care physician may prescribe a kidney transplant.

In what manner can kidney malady be counteracted?

Some hazard factors for kidney sickness —, for example, age, race, or family ancestry — are difficult to control. In any case, there are measures you can take to help anticipate kidney infection:

drink a lot of water

control glucose in the event that you have diabetes

control circulatory strain

lessen salt admission

stop smoking

Be cautious with over-the-counter medications

You ought to consistently adhere to the measurement guidelines for over-the-counter prescriptions. Taking an excessive amount of headache medicine (Bayer) or ibuprofen (Advil, Motrin) can cause kidney harm. Call your primary care physician if the ordinary portions of these meds aren't controlling your agony successfully.

Get tried

Get some information about getting a blood test for kidney issues. Kidney issues for the most part don't cause side effects until they're further developed. A fundamental metabolic board (BMP) is a standard blood test that should be possible as a component of a normal therapeutic test. It checks your blood for creatinine or urea. These are synthetic compounds that break into the blood when the kidneys aren't working appropriately. A BMP can distinguish kidney issues early, when they're simpler to treat. You ought to be tried every year on the off chance that you have diabetes, coronary illness, or hypertension.

Farthest point certain nourishments

Various synthetic compounds in your nourishment can add to specific kinds of kidney stones. These include:

inordinate sodium

creature protein, for example, meat and chicken citrus extract, found in citrus natural products, for example, oranges, lemons, and grapefruits oxalate, a substance found in beets, spinach, sweet potatoes, and chocolate

Get some information about calcium

Converse with your PCP before taking a calcium supplement. Some calcium enhancements have been connected to an expanded danger of kidney stones.

More About Kidney Diseases

Kidney malady can influence your body's capacity to clean your blood, sift additional water through of your blood, and help control your circulatory strain. It can likewise influence red platelet creation and nutrient D digestion required for bone wellbeing. You're brought into the world with two kidneys. They're on either side of your spine, simply over your midriff.

At the point when your kidneys are harmed, squander items and liquid can develop in your body. That can cause expanding in your lower legs, queasiness, shortcoming, poor rest, and brevity of breath. Without treatment, the harm can deteriorate and your kidneys may in the long run quit working. That is not kidding, and it tends to be hazardous.

What Your Kidneys Do

Sound kidneys:

Keep a parity of water and minerals, (for example, sodium, potassium, and phosphorus) in your blood. Expel squander from your blood after processing, muscle movement, and introduction to synthetic compounds or drugs. Make renin, which your body uses to help deal with your circulatory strain. Make a synthetic called erythropoietin, which prompts your body to make red platelets. Make a functioning type of nutrient D, required for bone wellbeing and different things

Intense Kidney Problems

In the event that your kidneys all of a sudden quit working, specialists call it intense kidney damage or intense renal disappointment. The fundamental driver are:

Conditions That Affect Your Kidneys

Your kidneys help channel all the waste items your body develops in its characteristic procedures. Gain more from WebMD about the medicinal issues that can hurt them.

Insufficient blood stream to the kidneys

Direct harm to the kidneys themselves

Pee sponsored up in the kidneys

Those things can happen when you:

Have horrendous damage with blood misfortune, for example, in an auto wreck

Are dried out or your muscle tissue separates, sending an excess of protein into your circulatory system

Go into stun on the grounds that you have a serious contamination called sepsis

Have an expanded prostate that hinders your pee stream

Ingest certain medications or are around sure poisons that straightforwardly harm the kidney

Have inconveniences during a pregnancy, for example, eclampsia and pre-eclampsia

Immune system sicknesses, when your insusceptible framework assaults your body, can likewise cause intense kidney damage. Individuals with extreme heart or liver disappointment usually go into intense kidney damage, also.

Interminable Kidney Disease

At the point when your kidneys don't function admirably for longer than 3 months, specialists call it constant kidney sickness. You might not have any manifestations in the beginning times, yet that is the point at which it's more straightforward to treat.

Ten Signs you might be having kidney diseases

In excess of 37 million American grown-ups are living with kidney illness and most don't have any acquaintance with it. "There are various physical indications of kidney infection, yet some of the time individuals ascribe them to different conditions. Additionally, those with kidney ailment tend not to encounter side effects until the exceptionally late stages, when the kidneys are falling flat or when there are a lot of protein in the pee. This is one reason why just 10% of individuals with incessant kidney malady realize that they have it," says Dr. Joseph Vassalotti, Chief Medical Officer at the National Kidney Foundation. While the best way to know without a doubt in the event that you have kidney infection is to get tried, Dr. Vassalotti shares 10 potential signs you may have kidney infection. In case you're in danger for kidney illness because of hypertension, diabetes, a family ancestry of kidney disappointment or in case you're more seasoned than age 60, it's essential to get tried every year for kidney infection. Make certain to specify any manifestations you're encountering to your social insurance expert. You're progressively worn out, have less vitality or are experiencing difficulty concentrating. An extreme abatement in kidney capacity can prompt a development of poisons and pollutions in the blood. This can make individuals feel worn out, frail and can make it difficult to focus. Another confusion of kidney sickness is frailty, which can cause shortcoming and exhaustion. You're experiencing difficulty resting. At the point when the kidneys aren't sifting appropriately, poisons remain in the blood as opposed to leaving the body through the pee. This can make it hard to rest. There is likewise a connection among corpulence and interminable kidney illness, and rest apnea is progressively regular in those with incessant kidney infection, contrasted and the all-inclusive community.

You have dry and irritated skin. Sound kidneys do numerous significant occupations. They expel squanders and additional liquid from your body, help make red platelets, help keep bones solid and work to keep up the perfect measure of minerals in your blood. Dry and bothersome skin can be an indication of the mineral and bone sickness that frequently goes with cutting edge kidney malady, when the kidneys are never again ready to keep the correct equalization of minerals and supplements in your blood.

You want to pee all the more regularly. In the event that you want to pee all the more regularly, particularly around evening time, this can be an indication of kidney sickness. At the point when the kidneys channels are harmed, it can make an expansion in the inclination pee. Some of the time this can likewise be an indication of a urinary disease or amplified prostate in men. You see blood in your pee. Sound kidneys commonly keep the platelets in the body when sifting squanders from the blood to make pee, however when the kidney's channels have been harmed, these platelets can begin to "spill" out into the pee.

Notwithstanding flagging kidney malady, blood in the pee can be demonstrative of tumors, kidney stones or a disease.

Your pee is frothy. Inordinate air pockets in the pee – particularly those that expect you to flush a few times before they leave—demonstrate protein in the pee. This froth may resemble the froth you see when scrambling eggs, as the basic protein found in pee, egg whites, is a similar protein that is found in eggs.

You're encountering relentless puffiness around your eyes. Protein in the pee is an early sign that the kidneys' channels have been harmed, enabling protein to spill into the pee. This puffiness around your eyes can be because of the way that your kidneys are releasing a lot of protein in the pee, as opposed to keeping it in the body.

Your lower legs and feet are swollen. Diminished kidney capacity can prompt sodium maintenance, causing expanding in your feet and lower legs. Growing in the lower furthest points can likewise be an indication of coronary illness, liver sickness and constant leg vein issues.

You have a poor hunger. This is an exceptionally broad side effect, however a development of poisons coming about because of diminished kidney capacity can be one of the causes.

Your muscles are cramping. Electrolyte uneven characters can result from hindered kidney work. For instance, low calcium levels and inadequately controlled phosphorus may add to muscle cramping.

Why does the renal diet work?

Renal diet works because the shape of the body along with the digestion is totally effective in this regard for the body and following are the steps that are followed for the better work of the renal diet.

Eating Right for Chronic Kidney Disease

You may need to change what you eat to deal with your ceaseless kidney illness (CKD). Work with an enlisted dietitian to build up a supper plan that incorporates nourishments that you appreciate eating while at the same time keeping up your kidney wellbeing.

The means underneath will assist you with eating directly as you deal with your kidney ailment. The initial three stages (1-3) are significant for all individuals with kidney ailment. The last two stages (4-5) may wind up significant as your kidney capacity goes down.

The initial steps to eating right

Stage 1: Choose and plan nourishments with less salt and sodium

Why? To help control your circulatory strain. You're eating regimen ought to contain under 2,300 milligrams of sodium every day. Purchase new nourishment frequently. Sodium (a piece of salt) is added to many arranged or bundled nourishments you purchase at the general store or at eateries. Cook nourishments without any preparation as opposed to eating arranged nourishments, "quick" nourishments, solidified meals, and canned food sources that are higher in sodium. At the point when you set up your very own nourishment, you control what goes into it.

Use flavors, herbs, and sans sodium seasonings instead of salt.

Check for sodium on the Nutrition Facts mark of nourishment bundles. A Daily Value of 20 percent or more means the nourishment is high in sodium. Attempt lower-sodium renditions of solidified meals and other comfort nourishments. Wash canned vegetables, beans, meats, and fish with water before eating.

Stage 2: Eat the perfect sum and the correct sorts of protein

Why? To help ensure your kidneys. At the point when your body utilizes protein, it produces squander. Your kidneys evacuate this waste. Eating more protein than you need may make your kidneys work more enthusiastically. Eat little parts of protein nourishments.

Protein is found in nourishments from plants and creatures. The vast majority eat the two kinds of protein. Converse with your dietitian about how to pick the correct mix of protein nourishments for you.

Creature protein nourishments:

Chicken

Fish

Meat

Eggs

Dairy

A cooked bit of chicken, fish, or meat is around 2 to 3 ounces or about the size of a deck of cards. A bit of dairy nourishments is ½ cup of milk or yogurt, or one cut of cheddar.

Plant-protein nourishments:

Beans

Nuts

Grains

A segment of cooked beans is about ½ cup, and a segment of nuts is ¼ cup. A bit of bread is solitary cut, and a part of cooked rice or cooked noodles is ½ cup.

Stage 3: Choose nourishments that are solid for your heart

Why? To assist keep with fatting from working up in your veins, heart, and kidneys. To assist keep with fatting from working up in your veins, heart, and kidneys.

Flame broil, sear, heat, dish, or pan-fried food nourishments, rather than profound fricasseeing.

Cook with nonstick cooking shower or a limited quantity of olive oil rather than spread.

Cut back excess from meat and expel skin from poultry before eating.

Attempt to constrain soaked and trans fats. Peruse the nourishment name.

Heart-solid nourishments:

Lean cuts of meat, for example, midsection or round

Poultry without the skin

Fish

Beans

Vegetables

Organic products

Low-fat or sans fat milk, yogurt, and cheddar

Farthest point liquor

Drink liquor just with some restraint: close to one beverage for each day on the off chance that you are a lady, and close to two in the event that you are a man. Drinking a lot of liquor can harm the liver, heart, and cerebrum and cause genuine medical issues. Ask your social insurance supplier how much liquor you can drink securely.

The subsequent stages to eating right

As your kidney capacity goes down, you may need to eat nourishments with less phosphorus and potassium. Your social insurance supplier will utilize lab tests to check phosphorus and potassium levels in your blood, and you can work with your dietitian to change your feast plan. More data is given in the NIDDK wellbeing point, Nutrition for Advanced Chronic Kidney Disease.

Stage 4: Choose nourishments and beverages with less phosphorus

Why? To help ensure your bones and veins. At the point when you have CKD, phosphorus can develop in your blood. A lot of phosphorus in your blood pulls calcium from your bones, making your bones slender, frail, and bound to break. Significant levels of phosphorus in your blood can likewise cause irritated skin, and bone and joint agony.

Many bundled nourishments have included phosphorus. Search for phosphorus—or for words with "PHOS"— on fixing names.

Shop meats and some new meat and poultry can have included phosphorus. Request that the butcher assist you with picking crisp meats without included phosphorus.

Nourishments Lower in Phosphorus

Crisp products of the soil

Breads, pasta, rice

Rice milk (not advanced)

Corn and rice oats

Light-hued soft drinks/pop, for example, lemon-lime or natively constructed frosted tea

Nourishments Higher in Phosphorus

Meat, poultry, fish

Wheat grains and cereal

Dairy nourishments

Beans, lentils, nuts

Dim shaded soft drinks/pop, fruit juice, some packaged or canned frosted teas that have included phosphorus

Your social insurance supplier may converse with you about taking a phosphate folio with dinners to bring down the measure of phosphorus in your blood. A phosphate fastener is a drug that demonstrations like a wipe to absorb, or tie, phosphorus while it is in the stomach. Since it is bound, the phosphorus doesn't get into your blood. Rather, your body expels the phosphorus through your stool.

Stage 5: Choose nourishments with the perfect measure of potassium

Why? To support your nerves and muscles work the correct way. Issues can happen when blood potassium levels are excessively high or excessively low. Harmed kidneys enable potassium to develop in your blood, which can cause genuine heart issues. Your nourishment and drink decisions can assist you with bringing down your potassium level, if necessary.

Salt substitutes can be exceptionally high in potassium. Peruse the fixing mark. Check with your supplier about utilizing salt substitutes.

Channel canned products of the soil before eating.

Nourishments Lower in Potassium

Apples, peaches

Carrots, green beans

White bread and pasta

White rice

Rice milk (not improved)

Cooked rice and wheat grains, corn meal

Apple, grape, or cranberry juice

Nourishments Higher in Potassium

Oranges, bananas, and squeezed orange

Potatoes, tomatoes

Dark colored and wild rice

Grain oats

Dairy nourishments

Entire wheat bread and pasta

Beans and nuts

A few drugs additionally can raise your potassium level. Your social insurance supplier may alter the meds you take.

What are renal diet benefits?

There are many benefits of renal diet as it bolsters vitamin C supplementation.

The significance of satisfactory nutrient C, or ascorbic corrosive, as a cell reinforcement and in collagen amalgamation is settled; be that as it may, there are extraordinary worries with respect to keeping away from over the top sums in CKD. Current proposals for support hemodialysis (MHD) patients exhort supplementation with ascorbic corrosive 75-90 mg every day (Nephrol Dial Transplant. 2007;22[Suppl 2]:ii45-ii87) to supplant the misfortunes of this water-dissolvable nutrient that happen during dialysis. This measure of nutrient C is found in most renal multivitamins, i.e., nutrient blends endorsed explicitly to require the necessities of MHD patients, however evaluates from the Dialysis Outcomes and Practice Patterns Study (DOPPS) demonstrate that renal multivitamins are recommended for just about

70% of dialysis patients in the United States (Am J Kidney Dis. 2004; 44[5 Suppl 2]:61-67).

With respect to advantages of renal multivitamin use, the creators report that "patients taking such nutrients had a 16% lower mortality hazard than patients not taking water-dissolvable nutrients, after modification for age, sex, race, comorbid conditions, hemoglobin, serum egg whites, weight record, time on HD, normal office single-pool Kt/V, and normal office standardized protein catabolic rate." Since dietary wellsprings of nutrient C are frequently limited in view of worries about potassium, an everyday renal multivitamin can be a significant piece of standard consideration for dialysis patients. Since nutrient C is discharged by the kidney, consumption more noteworthy than 100-200 mg/day ought to be stayed away from in CKD to maintain a strategic distance from oxalosis, which is the gathering of the metabolic result of ascorbic corrosive. Numerous organs and tissues of the body can be influenced by oxalate stores, including the kidneys. Instances of intense renal disappointment (ARF) have been reported. As of late, Nankivell and Murali detailed oxalosis bringing about unite disappointment in a kidney transplant beneficiary who had been taking self-endorsed dosages of nutrient C 2,000 mg every day as a dialysis tolerant for the three years before transplant (N Engl J Med. 2008;358:e4).

So also, a case report by McHugh and partners (Anaesth Intensive Care. 2008;36:585-588) portrays mortality from nutrient C-actuated ARF. Oxalosis was affirmed on post-mortem in this patient, who, unbeknownst to doctors, had been ingesting "a few grams for every day" of nutrient C in the conviction that it would be useful for his wellbeing.

Movement to renal parenchymal harm and end-organize renal illness, which is by all accounts to a great extent free of the underlying affront, is the last basic pathway for ceaseless, proteinuric nephropathies in creatures and people. The key occasion is upgraded glomerular hairlike weight; this weakens glomerular penetrability to proteins and licenses unreasonable measures of proteins to arrive at the lumen of the proximal tubule. The optional procedure of reabsorption of sifted proteins can add to renal interstitial damage by enacting intracellular occasions, including upregulation of the qualities encoding vasoactive and fiery go betweens. Both interstitial irritation and movement of malady can be constrained by such medications as angiotensin-changing over catalyst inhibitors, which reinforce the glomerular porousness obstruction to proteins and in this manner limit proteinuria and separated protein-subordinate provocative sign. Clinical information firmly propose that abatement would now be able to be accomplished in certain patients with constant renal infection. On account of the momentum slack time between beginning treatment and reduction, be that as it may, a significant extent of patients still progresses to end-arrange renal sickness before renal capacity starts to settle. A multimodal approach that focuses on lessening or evacuating all hazard components related with the movement of renal infection may diminish the opportunity to reduction of the ailment for most patients with proteinuric nephropathies.

Cardiovascular and renal advantages of dry bean and soybean consumption

Dry beans and soybeans are supplement thick, fiber-rich, and are top notch wellsprings of protein. Defensive and restorative impacts of both dry bean and soybean admission have been reported. Studies show that dry bean admission can possibly diminish serum cholesterol focuses, improve numerous parts of the diabetic state, and give metabolic advantages that guide in weight control. Soybeans are a novel wellspring of the isoflavones genistein and diadzein, which have various organic capacities. Soybeans and soyfoods conceivably have multifaceted wellbeing advancing impacts, including cholesterol decrease, improved vascular wellbeing, saved bone mineral thickness, and decrease of menopausal side effects. Soy seems to effectsly affect renal capacity, in spite of the fact that these impacts are not surely known. Though populaces devouring high admissions of soy have lower prevalences of specific malignancies, conclusive test information are deficient to explain a defensive job of soy. The accessibility of vegetable items and assets is expanding, fusing dry beans and soyfoods into the eating routine can be down to earth and pleasant. With the move toward a more plant-based eating routine, dry beans and soy will be powerful instruments in the treatment and aversion of incessant illness.

Benefits of Renal Diet

To build up if the advantage of angiotensin changing over compound inhibitor treatment in hindering dynamic diabetic renal damage is because of a particular intrarenal impact of the fundamental hypotensive impact, we examined the impact of long haul ramipril treatment on circulatory strain, glomerular filtration rate, and urinary protein discharge in streptozotocin-diabetic precipitously hypertensive rodents. The hypotensive impact of ramipril was counteracted by a high salt eating regimen, which didn't adjust the level of renal angiotensin changing over compound hindrance. Three weeks after uninephrectomy and enlistment of diabetes, rodents were apportioned to three gatherings. Gatherings 1 and 2 were given 1% NaCl, though bunch 3 was given water as drinking arrangement. Multi week later, bunches 2 and 3 got 0.4 mg/kg/day ramipril in their drinking arrangement, which was proceeded over a 2-month time span. Ramipril delivered a circulatory strain fall just in water-drinking rodents (bunch 3) in spite of a comparable decrease in plasma and renal angiotensin changing over compound movement in bunches 2 and 3. Salt-stacked rodents had a dynamic increment in urinary protein discharge over the span of study. Ramipril treatment forestalled an expansion in protein discharge just in creatures given water and with a decreased systolic pulse. Glomerular filtration rate was comparable in every one of the three gatherings. Ramipril treatment improved creature endurance autonomously of a decrease in circulatory strain or an impact on proteinuria. In spite of the fact that it is conceivable that angiotensin changing over catalyst inhibitors have explicit intrarenal impacts lessening movement of diabetic proteinuria, accompanying control of foundational circulatory strain has all the earmarks of being important to exhibit an advantage.

The renal benefits of a healthy life style

The renal advantages of a solid way of life Over the following decade, the quantity of patients with end-organize renal sickness requiring treatment by dialysis may twofold, and even created countries will experience issues adapting to this disturbing increment. There is a pressing need to feature the significance of modifiable hazard factors as a reason for treatment procedures to counteract the advancement and movement of constant kidney infection (CKD). This should incorporate dynamic augmentation of our present comprehension of a sound way of life.

Stoutness has turned into a universal plague, and adjusting this pestilence by changing way of life components is urgent to wellbeing and to the anticipation of kidney ailment today and later on. Liquor may effectsly affect renal capacity like those related with cardiovascular malady; nonetheless, liquor utilization is likewise a potential hazard factor for the advancement of glomerular harm, hypertension, and hypertensive nephrosclerosis. In patients with diabetes, smoking expands the danger of creating nephropathy and advancing to end-organize renal disappointment. Smoking likewise decreases renal capacity and builds albuminuria or proteinuria in the all-inclusive community. Dietary salt admission influences renal capacity through its consequences for pulse and fibrosis, perhaps by means of tumor development factor-β1–subordinate pathways, proposing that unnecessary salt admission might be a significant direct pathogenic factor for cardiovascular and renal ailment. Exercise decreases resting circulatory strain and avoids strange increments in pulse during physical effort. Humble weight reduction through diet and physical movement diminishes the frequency of type 2 diabetes in high-hazard people. The monetary weight forced by the expenses of dialysis and the high mortality identified with CKD presents a convincing contention for actualizing a savvy preventive methodology against end-arrange renal infection. To counteract CKD, proposals about a sound way of life went for the individual ought to be predictable with general wellbeing suggestions.

Interminable KIDNEY DISEASE AS AN EPIDEMIC PROBLEM

The overall increment in the quantity of patients with interminable kidney sickness (CKD) and subsequent end-organize renal ailment (ESRD) requiring renal substitution treatment is taking steps to arrive at pestilence extents throughout the following decade. ESRD profoundly affects grimness, mortality, and personal satisfaction, and forces a considerable weight on social insurance expenditure1. The scourge increment in the frequency of ESRD in numerous nations features the significance of the modifiable hazard factors as a reason for contriving treatment procedures to counteract the advancement and movement of CKD.

Endeavors to control the scourge of CKD and its cardiovascular difficulties have customarily centered around pharmacologic treatment of diabetes, hypertension, the lipid profile, and proteinuria2. CKD counteractive action and control systems incorporate characterizing in danger populaces and clarifying potential focuses for intercession. This should incorporate dynamic augmentation of our present comprehension of medicinal services and financial hazard factors.

Weight

Weight has turned into a universal plague, and there is developing understanding that specific way of life components is driving this pandemic. The cutting-edge way of life will in general support overconsumption and demoralizes consumption of vitality. Minor holes to be decided of vitality utilization and consumption lead to progressive yet enduring weight gain, and readdressing these patterns is essential to wellbeing and to counteracting kidney ailment today and in the future3.

The metabolic disorder, which is described by heftiness, insulin opposition, hyperinsulinemia, and dyslipidemia, might add to renal illness by numerous pathways, including the advancement of type 2 diabetes, hypertension, and cardiovascular malady. Corpulent patients can create proteinuria, which is trailed by dynamic loss of renal capacity in a generous extent of cases. Weight related glomerulopathy (ORG) is unmistakable from idiopathic central and segmental glomerulosclerosis (FSGS), and has a lower occurrence of nephrotic disorder, increasingly sluggish course, reliable nearness of glomerulomegaly, and milder foot process combination. The 10-overlay increment of ORG in rate in the course of recent years recommends a recently developing epidemic4.

Renal biopsies and post-mortem studies have indicated that FSGS causes the most well-known types of histologic injuries in corpulent patients with proteinuria. Extensive information show that hyperinsulinemia can intervene glomerular injury5, albeit glomerular hyperfiltration, hyperlipidemia, leptin, and resistin, a hormone discharged by adipocytes, may likewise be engaged with the pathogenesis of FSGS related with obesity6.

Weight reduction diminishes proteinuria in patients with ORG. Praga et al contemplated a gathering of patients with heftiness related proteinuria that was treated with hypocaloric abstains from food more than 1 year, and announced a mean weight reduction of 12% and a diminishing in proteinuria >80%7. In another investigation of 30 overweight patients, a mean weight reduction of 4% was trailed by a 31% diminishing in proteinuria8.

When all is said in done, being overweight is related with a 2-to 6-overlap increment in the danger of hypertension. Clinical preliminaries have additionally indicated that weight reduction is compelling in the essential avoidance of hypertension and in the decrease of both systolic and diastolic circulatory strain in patients with typical or high blood pressure9. Diminishing the pervasiveness of corpulence by improving way of life components should help in the essential counteractive action of CKD, especially in created nations. We tentatively concentrated a gathering of 35 beefy beyond belief patients (29 ladies and 6 men; mean weight file 47.6 ± 5.9 kg/m2) with stoutness related proteinuria who had been treated by biliopancreatic redirection.

Liquor

At present, epidemiologic examinations have revealed that moderate liquor and wine admission have defensive effects10. Liquor may helpfully influence renal capacity through comparable components to those revealed for cardiovascular illness, for example, by adjusting blood high-thickness lipoproteins, fibrinogen, insulin, and hemostatic elements. Burchfiel et al11 found that liquor admission was contrarily connected with a raised level of renal arteriolar hyalinization, autonomous of other cardiovascular hazard factors at post-mortem.

In any case, liquor may have both positive and negative consequences for renal capacity. Liquor utilization is a potential hazard factor for glomerular harm, hypertension, and hypertensive nephrosclerosis12. In exploratory examinations, liquor bolstered creatures have altogether lower renal capacity and more interstitial edema than their isocaloric controls13. A case-control concentrate dependent on self-reports found that normal utilization of in excess of 2 mixed beverages for each day was related with an expanded danger of kidney disappointment in the general population14. Interestingly, a forthcoming investigation of 1658 medical caretakers tried out the Nurses' Health Study found no relationship between moderate liquor utilization and pace of decrease in renal function15.

SMOKING AS A RENAL RISK FACTOR

Diabetologists were the first to perceive the unfavorable impacts of smoking on the kidney. In individuals with either type 1 or type 2 diabetes, smoking expands the danger of creating nephropathy and about pairs the pace of movement to end-arrange renal failure16. Smoking builds circulatory strain, tachycardia, convergences of catecholamines, and renovascular obstruction, which is joined by diminishes in glomerular filtration rate (GFR) and filtration portion. The impacts of smoking are ventured to be brought about by nicotine itself in light of the fact that these unfriendly impacts are not related with smoking sans nicotine cigarettes17. In subjects without renal infection, backhanded proof focuses to particular afferent vasoconstriction, which ought to ensure the glomerular microcirculation against the ascent in fundamental circulatory strain. Conversely, in patients with essential renal ailment, the intense increment in pulse isn't reliably joined by afferent vasoconstriction. It has been contended that in interminable smokers, compensatory initiation of nitric oxide–subordinate vasodilation neutralizes smoking-prompted vasoconstriction.

To research in the case of smoking is identified with albuminuria and unusual renal capacity in nondiabetic people, Pinto-Sietsma et al18 contemplated 7476 members in the Prevention of Renal and Vascular End Stage Disease Study. Current smokers ($\leq$20 or >20 cigarettes/day) and previous smokers had expanded middle egg whites discharge, and were bound to have high-ordinary albuminuria and microalbuminuria than nonsmokers. The level of members with a raised GFR was lower in previous smokers than in current smokers, and more prominent than in nonsmokers. Interestingly, the level of members with a diminished GFR was comparative in previous smokers and nonsmokers and fundamentally lower in previous smokers than in current smokers.

In a review case-control investigation of 4142 nondiabetic members 65 years old or more established in the Cardiovascular Health Study Cohort study, Bleyer et al19 found that the quantity of cigarettes smoked every day anticipated the decrease in renal capacity. This information propose that stopping smoking could diminish the danger of renal inadequacy in this more seasoned age gathering, which concurs with information from an investigation of 455 grown-ups in Minnesota that demonstrated that the reduction in creatinine freedom was more prominent in ex-smokers and ebb and flow smokers than in nonsmokers20. These examinations recommend that smoking decreases renal capacity and builds albuminuria or proteinuria in the all-inclusive community, a significant issue from a general wellbeing point of view.

Smoking is an incredible indicator of microalbuminuria in patients with essential hypertension. The commonness of microalbuminuria in lean, hypertensive smokers is almost twofold that in nonsmokers21. In an imminent investigation of variables anticipating the loss of renal capacity, Regalado et al22 distinguished smoking as the most dominant indicator in patients with essential hypertension however no proof of essential renal malady. Smoking may clarify at any rate some portion of the perception that patients with essential hypertension show a dynamic decay of renal capacity in spite of satisfactory control of blood pressure23.

Cigarette smoking speaks to a significant factor related with the movement of nephropathy in patients treated for hypertension and type 1 diabetes16. Absolutely, there are numerous valid justifications to quit smoking, especially for diabetic patients. Sawicki et al24 found that patients with type 1 diabetes and nephropathy who had great glycemic and circulatory strain control and had quit smoking had altogether lower danger of movement than current smokers. Male patients with glomerulonephritis25 or atherosclerotic ischemic nephropathy and who smoke26 are at expanded danger of hindered renal capacity.

Kasiske et al27 inspected the commonness and clinical connects of cigarette smoking in a huge accomplice of renal transplant beneficiaries. Contrasted and smoking under 25 pack-years or having never smoked, smoking in excess of 25 pack-years at transplantation was related with a 30% higher danger of join disappointment and an expanded danger of death. The impacts of smoking seem to disperse 5 years in the wake of stopping, recommending that more noteworthy exertion to urge patients to stop smoking before transplantation may diminish bleakness and mortality.

SALT INTAKE

The impact of salt on renal capacity is identified with both hypertension and to an immediate impact on renal capacity. Hypertension is both a reason and result of renal disappointment, yet the exact nature and commonness of hypertensive nephrosclerosis as a reason for renal disappointment stays disputable. There is solid proof that hypertension quickens the movement of exploratory renal infection and that control of pulse anticipates this movement. The connection between circulatory strain and ensuing renal infection gives off an impression of being certain and nonstop all through the full scope of pulse. In a 20-year network based, imminent, observational investigation of the relationship between hypertension on the future danger of CKD in 23,534 people, Haroun et al found a solid reviewed connection between CKD hazard and the Sixth Report of the Joint National Committee on Detection, Evaluation and Treatment of High Blood Pressure criteria for circulatory strain that was similarly solid in ladies as in men28.

Albeit epidemiologic information shows an immediate connection between dietary sodium admission and circulatory strain at the populace level, a few specialists question the all-inclusiveness of the discoveries and restrict general wellbeing proposals to diminish sodium consumption in the overall public. Results from creature ponders, epidemiologic examinations, and clinical preliminaries have demonstrated that a high admission of salt unfavorably influences circulatory strain. The DASH-Sodium preliminary tried the impacts on circulatory strain of 3 degrees of sodium: higher (focus of roughly 143 mmol/day, reflecting run of the mill U.S. utilization), middle of the road (focus of 106 mmol/day, mirroring the maximum furthest reaches of current U.S. suggestions), and lower (focus of 65 mmol/day). The information indicated that diminishing sodium admission diminished pulse in members with or without hypertension, which supports the present proposals to lower salt intake29,30.

A high salt admission might be applicable to the pathogenesis of fundamental hypertension and, free of its hypertensinogenic impacts, may create reactions in the kidney that lead to renal fibrosis, conceivably through expanded renal generation of tumor development factor (TGF)- β. Yu et al31 detailed the impact of a typical (1%) or high (8%) sodium chloride diet on myocardial and renal fibrosis in unexpectedly hypertensive rodents and normotensive Wistar-Kyoto rodents. High dietary salt prompted far reaching fibrosis and expanded TGF-β1 in the heart and kidney of normotensive and hypertensive rodents. These outcomes propose that dietary salt specifically affects fibrosis, conceivably by means of TGF-β1–subordinate pathways, and further recommend that over the top salt admission might be a significant direct pathogenic factor for cardiovascular and renal infection. Such information fortifies the present rules to constrain salt admission to 6 g/day.

PHYSICAL ACTIVITY

Inactive conduct is one of the most grounded hazard factors for some ceaseless illnesses and conditions, including cardiovascular sickness, hypertension, diabetes, heftiness, osteoporosis, colon malignant growth, renal infection, and sorrow. An ongoing audit of observational examinations announced that the hazard for all-cause mortality was 20% to 30% lower among grown-ups who met the Healthy People 2010 suggestions (30 minutes of moderate movement for at least 5 days of the week or 20 minutes of energetic action at least

3 times each week), and fairly lower for grown-ups who practiced tolerably or vivaciously at any rate a couple of times each month or once per week32.

Physical inertia is a significant hazard factor for cardiovascular ailment, and people who are less dynamic or physically fit have a 30% to half more serious hazard for hypertension. Together with diabetes mellitus, blood vessel hypertension is the most significant reason for renal disappointment and dialysis in created nations. The wellbeing and viability of gentle to direct exercise have noteworthy positive clinical ramifications for every single hypertensive patient. The activity actuated decrease in resting circulatory strain and counteractive action of irregular increments in pulse during physical effort lessens the danger of cardiovascular occasions. These progressions may likewise diminish the requirement for, and the expense and reactions of, antihypertensive medicine, and may improve personal satisfaction.

Easing back the movement of constant renal disappointment: Economic advantages and patients' points of view

In view of the anticipated increment in end-arrange renal malady (ESRD) rate (anticipated increment from 1998 to 2010; 86,825 to 172,667), pervasiveness (anticipated increment from 1998 to 2010; 326,217 to 661,330), and cost (complete cost dependent on 1998 proportion of Medicare versus non-Medicare cost; $16.74 billion of every 1998 to $39.35 billion out of 2010), a firm national exertion is expected to create procedures to slow the movement of constant renal disappointment (CRF). The inquiry emerges to how a lot of decrease in the movement of CRF would prompt an important reduction in the commonness and cost of ESRD. There are no target information that show the financial effect of easing back the movement of CRF. We built up a scientific model to evaluate the monetary effect of diminishing the movement of CRF by 10%, 20%, and 30%. US Renal Data System (USRDS) projections were utilized to demonstrate the pace of increment in ESRD frequency and pervasiveness. Glomerular filtration rate (GFR) at the commencement of ESRD treatment and cost per persistent year depended on USRDS information. The normal decrease in GFR in subjects with CRF was assessed to be 7.56 mL/min/y. All dollar reserve funds reflect 1998 expenses, limited for the future at 3% per annum. We likewise decided how a lot of easing back of the movement of CRF is significant from patients' points of view by methods for a composed survey (which asked about ability to go on a limited eating regimen, take six additional drugs for every day, and make six additional office visits for every year) and count of the pre-ESRD time picked up for various degrees of decrease in the movement of CRF. On the off chance that the pace of decrease in GFR diminished by 10%, 20%, and 30% after December 31, 1999, in all patients with GFRs of 60 mL/min or less, total direct human services investment funds through 2010 would approach roughly $18.56, $39.02, and $60.61 billion, individually. For a 10%, 20%, and 30% diminishing in the pace of decrease in GFR in all patients with a GFR of 30 mL/min or less, assessed total reserve funds through 2010 equivalent $9.06, $19.98, and $33.37 billion, separately. Reactions to the poll indicated that around 79% of subjects with CRF (n = 113) saw half a month's sans dialysis period noteworthy (P ≤ 0.0001), a period relating to a 10% decrease in the pace of decrease in GFR. Our information propose that the combined monetary effect of easing back the movement of CRF, even by as meager as 10%, would stun. They give solid help to the improvement and usage of concentrated reno-defensive endeavors starting at the beginning periods of constant renal illness and proceeded all through its course.

What you can eat and what is forbidden in the renal diet

Foods that are forbidden in the renal diet are as follows:

Dull Colored Colas

Notwithstanding the calories and sugar that colas give, they likewise contain added substances that contain phosphorus, particularly dull hued colas. Numerous nourishment producers include phosphorus during the preparing of nourishment and drinks to upgrade enhance, draw out timeframe of realistic usability and counteract staining. This additional phosphorus is significantly more absorbable by the human body than regular, creature or plant-based phosphorus (5Trusted Source). In contrast to common phosphorus, phosphorus as added substances isn't bound to protein. Or maybe, it's found as salt and exceptionally absorbable by the intestinal tract (6Trusted Source).

Added substance phosphorus can normally be found in an item's fixing rundown. Be that as it may, nourishment producers are not required to list the careful measure of added substance phosphorus on the nourishment mark. While added substance phosphorus substance changes relying upon the sort of cola, most dull hued colas are accepted to contain 50–100 mg in a 200-ml serving (7Trusted Source). Therefore, colas, particularly those dim in shading, ought to be evaded on a renal eating routine.

Avocados

Avocados are frequently touted for their numerous nutritious characteristics, including their heart-sound fats, fiber and cell reinforcements. While avocados are normally a sound expansion to the eating regimen, people with kidney infection may need to stay away from them. This is on the grounds that avocados are an exceptionally rich wellspring of potassium. One cup (150 grams) of avocado gives an astounding 727 mg of potassium (8). That is twofold the measure of potassium than a medium banana gives. In this way, avocados, including guacamole, ought to be kept away from on a renal eating routine, particularly on the off chance that you have been advised to watch your potassium admission.

Canned Foods

Canned nourishments, for example, soups, vegetables and beans, are regularly acquired as a result of their ease and comfort. Be that as it may, most canned nourishments contain high measures of sodium, as salt is added as an additive to build its timeframe of realistic usability (9Trusted Source). In view of the measure of sodium found in canned products, it's frequently prescribed that individuals with kidney ailment maintain a strategic distance from or limit their utilization.

Picking lower-sodium assortments or those named "no salt included" is ordinarily best. Also, depleting and flushing canned nourishments, for example, canned beans and fish, can diminish the sodium content by 33–80%, contingent upon the item

Entire Wheat Bread

Picking the correct bread can be mistaking for people with kidney ailment. Frequently for sound people, entire wheat bread is normally suggested over refined, white flour bread. Entire wheat bread might be a progressively nutritious decision, for the most part because of its higher fiber content. Be that as it may, white bread is typically suggested over entire wheat assortments for people with kidney sickness. This is a direct result of its phosphorus and potassium content. The more wheat and entire grains in the bread, the higher the phosphorus and potassium substance. For instance, a 1-ounce (30-gram) serving of entire wheat bread contains around 57 mg of phosphorus and 69 mg of potassium. In examination, white bread contains just 28 mg of both phosphorus and potassium (11, 12). Note that most bread and bread items, paying little heed to being white or entire wheat, additionally contain generally high measures of sodium (13Trusted Source). It's ideal to look at nourishment names of different sorts of bread, pick a lower-sodium choice, if conceivable, and screen your part estimates.

Dark colored Rice

Like entire wheat bread, dark colored rice is an entire grain that has a higher potassium and phosphorus content than its white rice partner. One cup of cooked darker rice contains 150 mg of phosphorus and 154 mg of potassium, while one cup of cooked white rice contains just 69 mg of phosphorus and 54 mg of potassium (14, 15). You might have the option to fit dark colored rice into a renal eating routine, yet just if the segment is controlled and offset with different nourishments to maintain a strategic distance from exorbitant every day admission of potassium and phosphorus. Bulgur, buckwheat, pearled grain and couscous are nutritious, lower-phosphorus grains that can make a decent substitute for dark colored rice.

Bananas

Bananas are known for their high potassium content. While they're normally low in sodium, one medium banana gives 422 mg of potassium (16). It might be hard to keep your every day potassium admission to 2,000 mg if a banana is a day by day staple. Shockingly, numerous other tropical organic products have high potassium substance also. Be that as it may, pineapples contain considerably less potassium than other tropical products of the soil be an increasingly appropriate, yet scrumptious, elective (17).

Dairy

Dairy items are plentiful in different nutrients and supplements. They're additionally a characteristic wellspring of phosphorus and potassium and a decent wellspring of protein. For instance, 1 cup (8 liquid ounces) of entire milk gives 222 mg of phosphorus and 349 mg of potassium (18). However, devouring an excessive amount of dairy, related to different phosphorus-rich nourishments, can be unfavorable to bone wellbeing in those with kidney sickness. This may sound astonishing, as milk and dairy are regularly prescribed for solid bones and muscle wellbeing. Be that as it may, when the kidneys are harmed, an excessive amount of phosphorus utilization can cause a development of phosphorus in the blood. This can make your bones slight and powerless after some time and increment the danger of bone breakage or crack (19Trusted Source). Dairy items are additionally high in protein. One cup (8 liquid ounces) of entire milk gives around 8 grams of protein (18).

Oranges and Orange Juice

While oranges and squeezed orange are seemingly most notable for their nutrient C substance, they are likewise rich wellsprings of potassium. One enormous orange (184 grams) gives 333 mg of potassium. Also, there are 473 mg of potassium in one cup (8 liquid ounces) of squeezed orange (20, 21). Given their potassium substance, oranges and squeezed orange likely should be maintained a strategic distance from or restricted on a renal eating routine. Grapes, apples and cranberries, just as their individual juices, are largely great substitutes for oranges and squeezed orange, as they have lower potassium substance.It might be critical to constrain dairy admission to dodge the development of protein squander in the blood. Dairy options like unenriched rice milk and almond milk are a lot of lower in potassium, phosphorus and protein than bovine's milk, making them a decent substitute for milk while on a renal eating routine.

What to eat in a renal diet?

Eat a high protein nourishment at each supper. This incorporates meat, fish, poultry, new pork or eggs.

Cut out potassium and phosphorus.

Dodge nutty spread, nut, seeds, dried beans and lentils. Despite the fact that these are high in protein, they are additionally high in potassium and phosphorous.

Utilize less salt and eat less salty nourishments. This may control pulse and lessen weight gains between dialysis sessions.

Use herbs, flavors and low-salt flavor enhancers instead of salt

Maintain a strategic distance from salt substitutes made with potassium.

Evade entire grain and high fiber nourishments, for example, entire wheat bread, grain oat and dark colored rice as far as possible your admission of phosphorous.

Utmost your admission of milk, yogurt and cheddar. These are high in phosphorus. Constraining dairy-based nourishments ensures your bones and veins.

All organic products have some potassium. Constraining potassium secures your heart. Pick apples and berries over oranges and bananas.

All vegetables have some potassium. Pick broccoli and cabbage over potatoes and asparagus.

What you can drink in the renal diet?

Things you can drink

How much liquid and kinds of liquid your admission is significant for the constant kidney infection patient to screen. A few patients may have been asked by their doctor to screen as well as limit the measure of liquids they take in.

Your liquid admission ought to be observed by inspecting your individual liquid status. In the event that you are holding liquid, cut back on your admission and the other way around.

1. Individuals with sound kidneys should drink 8-10 eight-ounce glasses (64 ounces) of water ordinary

2. Patients on dialysis as well as patients experiencing a "wiped out period," may display indications of lack of hydration. Indications of lack of hydration include: migraines,

indigestion, joint and back torment, kidney stones, clogging, exhaustion and dazedness.

3. Patients on diuretics might be progressively vulnerable to lack of hydration.

4. Drinking water brings down danger of urinary tract and bladder contaminations, which can be basic in kidney illness patients.

5. Indications of liquid over-burden incorporate swollen fingers and lower legs, hypertension, swelling and trouble relaxing.

Is liquor or soft drink awful for the kidneys?

Not generally. With some restraint, liquor and soft drink are not awful for the kidneys. Yet, both influence the kidneys in a roundabout way. Mixed refreshments and soft drinks are high in calories, and a lot of them are bad for anybody with diabetes. Diabetes is the main source of kidney disappointment. Likewise, while liquor influences the liver all the more straightforwardly, it can raise circulatory strain.

What's more, cause lack of hydration. Hypertension may harm the kidneys. Hypertension is the number two reason for kidney disappointment. Liquor likewise can be hazardous to drink when you are on certain sorts of medication. Try to get some information about how liquor can influence your medications.

Another investigation connected drinking at least two sugary beverages every day with an expanded hazard for hypertension.

Is cranberry squeeze useful for the kidneys?

Cranberry juice may help avoid urinary tract contaminations (UTIs). The juice makes it hard for germs (microscopic organisms) to develop in your bladder. In the event that you are inclined to UTI's as well as kidney contaminations, incorporating 100% cranberry squeeze in your day by day admission may be a smart thought.

Shouldn't something be said about caffeinated drinks?

Caffeinated beverages ought to be utilized with alert. They are soda pops whose makers promote that they support vitality. Most contain a wellspring of caffeine as their significant fixing. Interminable kidney sickness patients should screen the measure of caffeine that they incorporate into their weight control plans and limit it to under 200-mg/day. Allude to the rundown beneath for caffeine admission in like manner drinks and nourishment things.

Nourishment Item (Caffeine Content)

Blended Coffee (100mg)

Hershey's Milk Chocolate Kisses (5mg)

M&M's Milk Chocolate (16mg)

Mountain Dew (56mg)

Snapple Iced Tea (38mg)

Starbucks Coffee Frappuccino (166mg)

How much water would it be advisable for me to drink?

You should not have to drink eight glasses of water each day to remain sound, as once thought. Yet, water is as yet a superior decision than drinks that have caffeine like pop, espresso or tea. These beverages can really make you thirstier. Staying away from extra sugary squeezes and fruit juices is likewise a smart thought, particularly on the off chance that you have diabetes. Drinking a lot of water may likewise help avoid kidney stones. Continuously make a point to remain inside your doctor's liquid admission suggestions and watch for liquid over-burden.

Recipes

This chapter will throw light on various meals that have a renal ingredient in them

Breakfast

Dilly Scrambled Eggs

Ingredients

2 huge eggs

1/8 teaspoon dark pepper

1 teaspoon dried dill weed

1 tablespoon disintegrated goat cheddar

Supplements per serving

Calories 194

Protein 16 g

Starches 1 g

Fat 14 g

Cholesterol 434 mg

Sodium 213 mg

Potassium 192 mg

Phosphorus 250 mg

Calcium 214 mg

Fiber 0.2 g

Readiness

Beat the eggs in a bowl; empty them into a nonstick skillet over medium warmth.

Include dark pepper and dill weed to eggs.

Cook until eggs are mixed.

Top with disintegrated goat cheddar before serving.

Renal and renal diabetic nourishment decisions

2 meat

1 fat

Sugar decisions

Supportive insights

1/2 cup low cholesterol egg item can be substituted for 2 eggs for a lower fat and cholesterol dish. Cholesterol is diminished to 11 mg, fat 4 mg, and phosphorus 73 mg.

Cindy inclines toward The Pampered Chef® All-Purpose Dill Mix.

Substitute one tablespoon crisp dill for dried dill weed whenever wanted.

Speedy and Easy Apple Oatmeal Custard

Fixings

1/3 cup snappy cooking oats

1 enormous egg

1/2 cup almond milk

1/4 teaspoon cinnamon

1/2 medium apple

Supplements per serving

Calories 248

Protein 11 g

Sugars 33 g

Fat 8 g

Cholesterol 186 mg

Sodium 164 mg

Potassium 362 mg

Phosphorus 240 mg

Calcium 154 mg

Fiber 5.8 g

Planning

Center and finely slash apple half.

Join oats, egg and almond milk in a huge mug. Mix well with a fork. Include cinnamon and apple. Mix again until completely blended. Cook in microwave on high for 2 minutes. Lighten with a fork. Cook an extra 30 to 60 seconds if necessary. Mix in somewhat more milk or water if more slender oat is wanted.

Renal and renal diabetic nourishment decisions

1 meat

1 starch

1 milk substitute

1 organic product, low potassium

Sugar decisions

2

Supportive clues

For extra flavor supplant ground cinnamon with finely ground stick cinnamon.

Cooking time may change for various microwaves.

Sprinkle oats with 2 teaspoons of nectar whenever wanted. Consider an extra 12 grams of starch and 1 sugar decision in the event that you pursue a starch tallying dinner plan for diabetes. Substitute 1/4 cup 1% low fat milk and 1/4 cup water for almond milk whenever liked. These progressions the protein to 12 grams, phosphorus to 278 mg and potassium to 358 mg.

Oats is higher in potassium and phosphorus contrasted with refined grains, however can be incorporated into most kidney abstains from food. Talk about with your dietitian on the off chance that you are uncertain.

Microwave Coffee Cup Egg Scramble

Fixings

1 enormous egg

2 enormous egg whites

2 tablespoons 1% low fat milk

1/8 teaspoon dark pepper

Supplements per serving

Calories 117

Protein 15 g

Starches 3 g

Fat 5 g

Cholesterol 188 mg

Sodium 194 mg

Potassium 226 mg

Phosphorus 138 mg

Calcium 72 mg

Fiber 0 g

Arrangement

Splash a 12-ounce espresso mug with cooking shower. Consolidate the milk, egg and egg whites in the mug and beat until mixed. Spot espresso mug in microwave and cook for 45 seconds; expel and mix. Microwave an expansion 30-45 seconds, until eggs are nearly set.

Sprinkle with pepper and appreciate.

Need increasingly heavenly kidney-accommodating plans like Microwave Coffee Cup Egg Scramble?

Smoothies and drinks

Blueberry Smoothie

Fixings

1 cup solidified blueberries

8 bundles of Splenda®

6 tablespoons of protein powder

8 ice 3D squares

14 ounces of squeezed apple (no additional sugar)

Supplements per serving

Calories 108

Protein 9 g

Starches 18 g

Fat 0 g

Cholesterol 0 mg

Sodium 27 mg

Potassium 183 mg

Phosphorus 42 mg

Calcium 57 mg

Fiber 1.2 g

Arrangement

Spot all fixings in a blender and mix until smooth.

Simple Pineapple Protein Smoothie

Fixings

3/4 cup pineapple sherbet or sorbet

1 scoop vanilla whey protein powder

1/2 cup water

2 ice 3D squares, discretionary

Supplements per serving

Calories 268

Protein 18 g

Starches 40 g

Fat 4 g

Cholesterol 36 mg

Sodium 93 mg

Potassium 237 mg

Phosphorus 160 mg

Calcium 160 mg

Fiber 1.4 g

Arrangement

In a blender, include pineapple sherbet, whey protein powder and water (ice 3D squares discretionary).

Promptly mix for 30 to 45 seconds.

Snacks and sides

Nibbling when you're on the kidney diet

Eating is alright on the kidney diet as long as you settle on solid decisions. As opposed to eating nourishment that is high in sodium, for example, a little sack of potato chips, a superior choice is a bit of kidney-accommodating organic product. You likewise need to think about the amount you eat by and large. Eating shouldn't be synonymous with blame. On the off chance that your doctor urges you to build your calorie admission, your renal dietitian will examine the best nibble decisions for you. Bites can compensate for low-calorie consumption when your hunger isn't so extraordinary.

Kidney-accommodating snacks at the supermarket

Experience any treat or wafer passageway of your neighborhood market and you'll locate a wide cluster of tidbits. In any case, on the off chance that you have CKD you should restrain or stay away from specific fixings that might be available in nibble nourishments. Your primary care physician or dietitian may prescribe that you limit your admission of phosphorus, potassium, sodium and calcium if your kidneys are never again ready to keep these minerals in balance. By instructing yourself and with the assistance of your social insurance group, there are numerous kidney-accommodating, sound and scrumptious snacks accessible. Go to the produce area where you can discover kidney-accommodating nourishments for a decent nibble choice. Here are a few nourishments useful for kidney wellbeing:

Apples

Blueberries

Carrot sticks

Fruits

Dried, improved cranberries

Grapes

Raspberries

Red ringer peppers

Red leaf lettuce

Strawberries

Lunch

Bar-b-que Chicken Pita Pizza

Fixings

2 pita breads, 6-1/2" size

3 tablespoons low-sodium grill sauce

1/4 cup purple onion

2 tablespoons disintegrated feta cheddar

4 ounces chicken, cooked

1/8 teaspoon garlic powder

Supplements per serving

Calories 320

Protein 23 g

Sugars 37 g

Fat 9 g

Cholesterol 55 mg

Sodium 523 mg

Potassium 255 mg

Phosphorus 221 mg

Calcium 163 mg

Fiber 2.4 g

Planning

Preheat broiler to 350° F.

Shower preparing sheet with nonstick cooking splash and spot 2 pitas on sheet.

Spread 1-1/2 tablespoon BBQ sauce on every pita.

Hack onion and spread over pitas.

3D square chicken and spread over pitas.

Sprinkle feta cheddar and garlic powder over pitas.

Prepare for 11 to 13 minutes.

Conclusion

To conclude the book, you have to be very careful about diet intakes that you do throughout your routine. You need to be curious about every calorie that goes in you. You have been provided with all the reasons in this book about the process of renal diet. Renal diet can give you a healthy ph and can avert any harmful stroke of acidity in the body. Acidity can be dangerous in profuse accumulation fats, rise to inflammatory disease, the rupture in many digestion organs and having a rusted metabolism that does not work in the flow. On the contrary, renal diet can give you a fresh intake of all healthy diets that can be very healthy and caring for you. These diets are present in all formats.

They are in breakfast recipes, the dinner recipes, the lunch recipes, the smoothies and the sweat desserts that can up-satisfaction in your mouth. You do not have to be an expert of medicine to know which diet to follow when. You just have to know the diet intake of your own body and see how you are able to cater to the plight of diseases. You must not be able to compound yourself with the attack of acidity but must have the courage to use these diets and recover at the earliest.

These diets have everything in their DNA. They have the minerals, the enzymes, the protein, the amino acids, and whatnot. Green refluxes along with curing liquids are present in these diets and they come in all whims and fancies of the diet expression. There is no rocket science behind their creation and one has to be very intelligent while creating them. You can also follow this book and will get a splendid amount of results in no time. It is available at an affordable price.

Try your best in avoiding any acidic diet at all cost even if it gives you a great amount of relish. The idea is fats and mineral are very delicious but they come with devious outcomes of fat accumulation and strengths.

You need to understand that long aging is only possible if you have a balanced diet intake and this diet can be only of an keto.

To make conclusive remarks of the book about the benefits of an renal diet, the first and foremost is the sheer activeness that a person tends to achieve while he is eating an renal diet. He feels healthy and looks healthy and wants to be doing a lot of things while he is having an renal diet. He can think properly and can get rid of inflammatory diseases that can cause him suffering. He has a strong discipline that can be navigated in any way possible and thus, he is the next big thing for his users. Also, the longevity of life in this scenario and truly, an renal diet can do a lot of wonders for the individual. Therefore, an renal diet has a lot to do for the fitness and active-ness in the human body.

Furthermore, If you want to look green and fresh on your face, then the renal diet can be very helpful in this regard. Studies show that the renal diet is very popular in making a healthy face for you. The number of herbs and breakfast recipes you have for yourself, up-bring a good amount of freshness on your face as well on your skin. Thus, renal diet is very crucial for having great skin and face.

An renal diet protects bone density and muscle mass. The mineral intake that you get after having an renal diet can protect your bone density. The bones need certain minerals that are used to cure the excessive number of hurdles one gets while running. The minerals are given by the renal diet and you are able to get a stronger bone for life. If you are a bodybuilder and want to reap the benefits of the bone then you have to accumulate more renal diet in you that can be very beneficial for you. The muscle mass can be secured in an acute manner if you tend to get more and more almonds and other renal dietaries. You have to be very lenient when you are having the renal diet because the benefit of an renal diet like the muscle mass and the bone density will be instrumental for you. Just always look at the bright side of the diet and you will feel very productive while you do it.

In today's world, tensions are like a haunting disease that wants to remain at your back for no reason. Everywhere you go, you get a tertiary level of tension. There is the tension of graduating, the tension of succeeding in life, the tension of getting a job and tension of whatnot. You believe that tension can be very successive for you but in the latter, it turns out to be adverse. Scientists have claimed very medical drugs for its cure but the only reasonable cure for are the use of an renal diet. The enzymes that you get through vegetables lower the risk of your hyper blood tension and then you can achieve all the relish of your lifestyle in no time. Also, your blood level starts to resonate with full capacity and you will feel like a superman every place you go, therefore; hypertension and tensed matters get an upper hand of resolution when you get to know the prospect of an renal diet.

You are able to get a lot of chronic pains in your body due to many reasons. You get to the bottom of any problem; you solve it and end up having chronic pain in your body. Chronic pain refers to any tertiary amount of pain in your body and you are able to get to the harmfulness of it in no time. Therefore, chronic pain is the most devastating headache that you can get and the only effective cure of it is the renal diet. Yes, the renal diet is very important for you to maintain as the blood level minimizes when lemon or other keto water is induced in the body. So, this is another benefit of an renal diet and it does not matter if you are a walker, a boxer or even a corporate worker, you must have an renal diet in you if you wish to give all that you crave.

In the end, we will only assure you good health and being a beginner, you must waste any further time and order this book in a jiffy.

Because health is wealth nobody became rich while being lazy and stubborn. This book is all that you need and you must get at all cost.